KIAC

NOV -- 2019

Praise for *The Yoga Plate*

"Tamal and Victoria have brought the awareness of yoga into our kitchens—the true foundational element that has the capability to level up the spiritual awareness in our food and touch the soul. *The Yoga Plate* brings compassion and right living for the benefit of our families, our planet, and our animals—a beautiful offering for good all around."

JULIE PIATT AND RICH ROLL
bestselling authors, wellness leaders,
chefs, and podcast hosts

"I love the way Victoria and Tamal introduce the philosophy of yoga as it is reflected on our plates. All of the recipes are designed according to the concept of *ahimsa*, or non-harm, which is part of the Eight Limb Path in yoga. I can't wait to try all of the recipes in the book and share them with my friends and family as they start to realize our eating choices are making a huge impact on the planet. Thank you, Tamal and Victoria, for making vegan cuisine fun, easy, and delicious."

KOYA WEBB
holistic health coach, yoga instructor,
and author of *Let Your Fears Make You Fierce*

"*The Yoga Plate* carries an important message, as well as practical tools (i.e. delicious recipes!) for truly living yoga as a lifestyle. It offers its readers a deeper pathway into peace, health, and harmony in our lives that comes from the holistic approach to yoga that it espouses."

KIMBERLY SNYDER, CN
New York Times bestselling author of *Recipes for Your Perfectly
Imperfect Life*, nutritionist, and founder of Solluna

"I'm a fan of Victoria and Tamal . . . they live their talk in spirit, in the work they do, and in the food they prepare. The food they make is clean, healthy, and so very delicious. Every morsel is always awesome. In my book, they are stars."

MIMI KIRK
bestselling author, raw food chef,
and international speaker

"Victoria showed us that vegan cooking and food could be fun, delicious, and totally doable! She was laid back and breezy and showed us that mindfulness with our food could be a pleasure and not a chore. We highly recommend incorporating her recipes and techniques into your lifestyle. You won't be disappointed!"

RYAN BATHE AND STERLING BROWN
stars of *This Is Us*

"Tamal and Victoria Dodge are some of the OGs of plant-based cooking and wellness. I did my 200-hour yoga teacher training with Tamal and always get teary-eyed speaking of his soulful teachings. His classes are transformative, kind, and connected. These two lead their lives from a place of authenticity and truth. I can't wait to get my hands on this book!"

SOPHIE JAFFE
owner of Philosophie Superfoods

"Some of my fondest memories are of hanging out with Tamal and Victoria in their kitchen and studio. If everyone could eat Victoria's homemade granola and listen to Tamal sing everyday, the world would be a better place. Amazing people = better world. They are such a huge part of that equation."

KATHRYN BUDIG
bestselling author, podcast host,
and international yoga instructor

"Tamal and Victoria Dodge are the living embodiment of the true yogic lifestyle. Their authenticity, knowledge, and expertise—not only in the area of nutrition, but in yoga philosophy, meditation, and compassionate living—are a rare gift in this world. I have no doubt *The Yoga Plate* will be of benefit to millions on the path to greater physical, mental, and spiritual health."

LIZ ARCH
author, international yoga teacher,
and *Yoga Journal* cover girl

the yoga plate

the yoga plate

Bring Your Practice into the Kitchen
with 108 Simple & Nourishing Vegan Recipes

TAMAL & VICTORIA DODGE

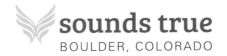
sounds true
BOULDER, COLORADO

Sounds True
Boulder, CO 80306

This book is not intended as a substitute for the medical recommendations of physicians, mental health professionals, or other health-care providers. Rather, it is intended to offer information to help the reader cooperate with physicians, mental health professionals, and health-care providers in a mutual quest for optimal well-being. We advise readers to carefully review and understand the ideas presented and to seek the advice of a qualified professional before attempting to use them.

Published 2019

Cover design by Rachael Murray
Book design by Beth Skelley

Original photography © 2019 Victoria Dodge

Printed in South Korea

Library of Congress Cataloging-in-Publication Data

Names: Dodge, Tamal, author. | Dodge, Victoria, author.
Title: The yoga plate : bring your practice into the kitchen with 108 simple
  & nourishing vegan recipes / Tamal and Victoria Dodge.
Description: Boulder, CO : Sounds True, [2019] | Includes index.
Identifiers: LCCN 2018057067 (print) | LCCN 2018057490 (ebook) |
  ISBN 9781683643517 (ebook) | ISBN 9781683643500 (hardback)
Subjects: LCSH: Vegan cooking. | One-dish meals. | LCGFT: Cookbooks.
Classification: LCC TX837 (ebook) | LCC TX837 .D587 2019 (print) |
  DDC 641.5/6362—dc23
LC record available at https://lccn.loc.gov/2018057067

10 9 8 7 6 5 4 3 2 1

contents

our yoga journey

Our story is relatable, unique, different, and common all at the same time.

When we started dating in 2006, Tamal always suggested that we eat at a local plant-based restaurant. Halfway joking, Victoria finally asked, "Are we *ever* going to eat anywhere else?" This light comment triggered a potential deal breaker of a discussion as Tamal explained to Victoria his beliefs surrounding food and its importance in his life.

It might sound like Tamal was being a bit rigid, but for him, eating has always been meaningful and intentional . . . probably more so than it is for the average American. Born into a family that ran a yoga ashram, Tamal was raised to view food and eating as an extension of a yogic, meditative lifestyle. He was raised to abide by the concept of *ahimsa*—to do no harm—in all facets of his life. In fact, he has never in his entire life eaten meat, fish, or eggs, because all

of these foods require inflicting harm. Life in the ashram was treated as a moving meditation: every single meal, task, and interaction was completed mindfully and with the intention to relink with God. In other words, *everything* was viewed as yoga, with the postures he practiced on his mat being the least essential element of all.

A Wisconsin native, bred on cheese, meat, and potatoes and with a deer head proudly placed above the mantel in her childhood home, Victoria was taken aback. As luck would have it, right after this discussion she set off to join her parents in Florida for a family vacation. One night, Victoria and her dad went out to get grouper for dinner, which they always loved eating together. When their meal arrived, she excitedly dug in—only to find that the fish was rotten. Disgusted but not deterred, Victoria and her dad tried for a redo a few nights later. Once again, the grouper was bad. "Is this a sign?" she couldn't help but wonder.

"Okay, I'm willing to try this plant-based thing," Victoria told Tamal a few days later. Peering into her sparsely populated refrigerator, stocked only with milk, yogurt, and eggs, Tamal knew Victoria was in for a challenge.

Today, life couldn't be more different. Gone are the days of a dairy-laden refrigerator and meat-based dinners. Instead, Victoria and Tamal's entire family enjoys a delicious plant-based diet, jam-packed with greens and whole foods.

Not only has Victoria's diet changed, but so too has her philosophy about both food and life in general. It bears mentioning that before converting to a vegan lifestyle, she did lead a healthy life. However, food was more of an afterthought, and Victoria didn't have a baseline from which to understand how much better she could feel physically, mentally, and spiritually. Ten years later, she relishes preparing and enjoying meals as part of a meditative lifestyle, geared toward both spiritual and physical wellness. She feels more vibrant, grounded, and connected to her own self, the world around her, and the Supreme Soul.

So although we came to food in different ways and from different backgrounds, we found a common ground through yoga as it taught us the meaning of life and the path to helping others. We eat a whole-food, plant-based yoga diet that carries a deep spiritual undertone reflected by a specific lifestyle, which is what we're sharing in this book. We have been living a yoga life since we met and have continued to do so as our family grew, developing our practices and sharing the profound translations of ancient writings with those around us along the way.

This cookbook is more than a collection of recipes. It is a lifestyle book about how to turn every day into a spiritually infused meditation. This book is like a map, one readers can follow to alter their perception of the world and those around them. We encourage you to adopt a positive and joy-filled existence and a calm demeanor. This will be reflected in your internal landscape.

We have raised our children to explore yoga on a deeper level beyond yoga poses, to embrace yogic teachings, and to add these principles to their lives. If our kids can see the immense benefits of yoga, then we are pretty sure that people all over the world can take a little wisdom from this ancient science and incorporate it into their lives as well.

The recipes in *The Yoga Plate* are delicious and healthy, and they are grounded in yoga's most pure and sacred teachings, supporting a harmonious and tranquil existence. In this book, you'll find recipes and family tips that we accumulated and developed over the last ten years. This book is a labor of love for readers to enjoy. We hope you flourish in its lessons and take away a newfound path to living soulfully. Our little family is excited to share simple, easy, healthy dishes that are bound to become staples in your household.

We know how challenging it can be to cook something that nourishes the body, heals the mind, and fills the soul as well. So we have taken into consideration our busy lifestyles and the fact that many of us live in an urban landscape. When things are chaotic around us, it is refreshing to mindfully (but often quickly) make foods that will satisfy and energize.

The Yoga Plate is a collection of recipes lovingly and thoughtfully handpicked to share. But it is also a guide to grounding oneself, whatever one's living situation might be. The message of this book is to take ancient traditions and use them in modern applications. The results are a healthy body and peace of mind.

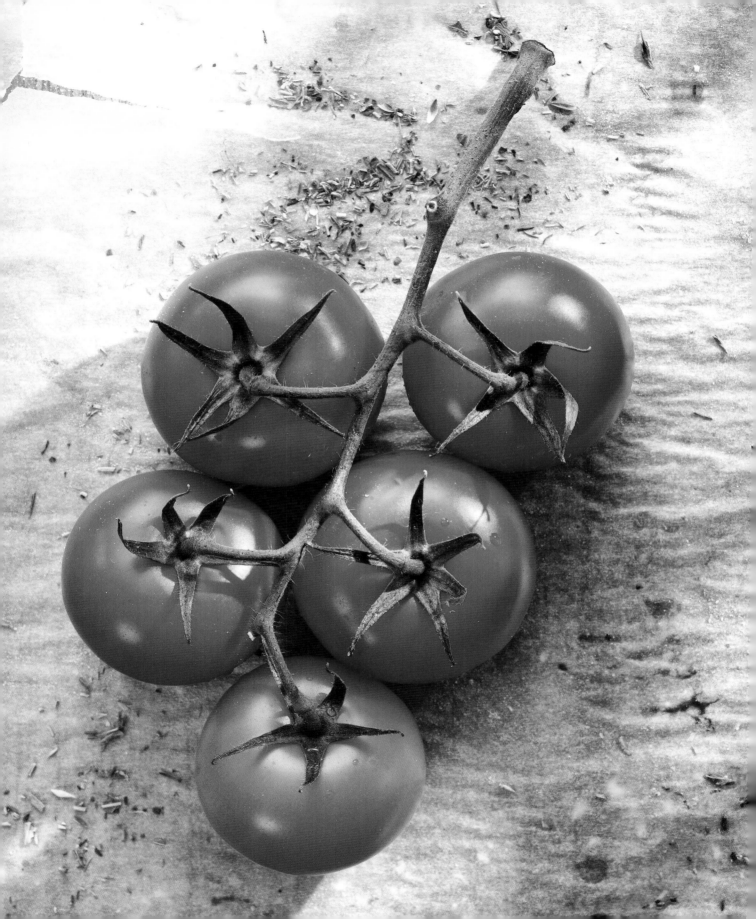

the yoga kitchen

If one offers Me with love and devotion a leaf,
a flower, fruit, or water, I will accept it.
BHAGAVAD GITA AS IT IS 9:26

off the mat, into the kitchen

For humanity to evolve spiritually, this diet is essential.

More than 36 million Americans today practice yoga. To be specific, more than 36 million people today practice the *physical postures* of yoga, known as *asana*. Talk to the vast majority of these asana practitioners, and they'll tell you that yoga has in some way bettered their lives, whether it be physically, mentally, emotionally, or spiritually.

But what so many of these 36 million Americans don't realize is that they are experiencing only the tip of the iceberg in their yoga practice. In fact, asana is just one of the Eight Limbs of Yoga as set forth by yogic master Patanjali in the Yoga Sutras circa 400 CE. However, in India, the birthplace of yoga, talk to the 99 percent of the country's population who are yogis, and they will tell you that asana is the least essential of their yoga practices. There, far more attention is placed on the philosophy of yoga than on the physicality of it. Without embedding the philosophy of yoga into its physical practice, Western yogis are missing out on so much.

Yoga is about far more than spending an hour on a rubber mat. It is about creating a spiritual life by transforming our daily activities into actions infused with a higher consciousness. That said, yoga is not a religion; it is nonsectarian and nondenominational. The path of yoga is about taking our lifestyle and moving it into a realm that harmonizes our will with the highest source.

The word *yoga* translates as "yoke." By definition, the ultimate goal of yoga is to yoke together—or create union—between the soul and our higher source by infusing our daily activities with spiritual intention and mindfulness.* By design, then, yoga is a prescription for a complete lifestyle that leads practitioners to a better, more whole and peaceful way of living. They are more connected to themselves; more connected to their bodies, to their minds, hearts, and souls; to other life on this planet; to the environment; and to the Supreme Soul. Asana is the gateway, yes—but there's so much more to explore.

How we eat is a key component in all of this because it represents both how we treat and nourish ourselves and how we view and care for the world and resources around us. We can make food choices that support us in both specific and holistic ways in body, mind, and spirit. Until now, there has yet to be a modern book that sets forth the correlation between yoga as a holistic practice, the dietary decisions we make, and the mind-set with which we view and eat food. With yoga now widely practiced throughout the United States, the time is ripe to introduce readers to the next level of their practice, so that they can take their yoga beyond just their mat and onto their plate.

Our modern culture is more technologically advanced than ever before. Yet at the same time, we have regressed in our ability to sustain the environment around us. It would seem like an oxymoron to say we are advanced but also primitive in our society, yet this truth is unfolding before our very eyes. According to the yoga system, the reason for such rise and decline is that we are indifferent when it comes to looking at the existence of the soul and our own spiritual well-being. You see, the more we rely on our senses and material perception, the more we may gain materially, but on the flip side we drastically decline spiritually.

Yoga teaches us that our senses are limited and that we shouldn't rely on them for the answers to life. For example, if we are in the desert and in the distance we think we see water and decide to chase after it, we get there only to discover it was a mirage. Our senses tricked us—we couldn't decipher what was real and what was fake.

. . . .

* Just a note: God is called many names: Rama, Yahweh, Jehovah, Gopala, Allah, Krishna, and so on. In the Yoga Sutras, Patanjali refers to God as Ishvara, which means "Supreme Soul." To honor the yoga system, we will be referring to God as the Supreme Soul throughout this book. However, you should refer to the higher source in whatever way feels most comfortable to you. After all, the main point is to create a personal connection between ourself and our higher source.

The yoga system encourages us to go beyond what our eyes, noses, ears, touch, and taste can tell us and move into a life filled with spiritual practice that takes us past the confines of the temporary material body. When we engage our mind and senses in spiritual rigor, we purify our consciousness, bringing us to a state of pure clarity and unselfish, magnanimous behavior. We start to look at the world differently, and we treat the world and all its living entities with kindness, compassion, and love.

The culture of today is telling us to eat more, buy more, enjoy more, and take in as much excess as possible before we die. Our culture has spun so far out of control that we are trying to enjoy material life at any cost, regardless of the impact on others and the world. We have put so much emphasis on living the material dream that we have lost sight of anything suggestive of spiritual consciousness.

When we believe we are material beings living in a material world, we tend to treat our planet like a landfill, without much regard for the future of everyone. But when we know that we are spiritual beings living in a material world and it is our duty to elevate our consciousness and those around us, then we start making progress in huge leaps and bounds. We want to create a minimal carbon footprint while leaving a huge spiritual exclamation point at the end of our road. Then we know that we have been of service to the planet and used our bodies wisely.

We are on such a fast track in our society that we don't realize how much harm we are doing even with the food we eat. We are told to consume hamburgers, milkshakes, pizza, and junk food, which is bad not only for our bodies but for our whole ecosystem. Even fad diets that may appear healthy can have a negative effect on the planet's resources. Our dietary habits cause astronomical amounts of damage to the world around us.

Yoga teaches us to examine and question life, to search our hearts and minds regularly, and to use our intellect for spiritual study and growth. And what better place to start than with the food we eat? The information and advertisements we take in do not put the planet and spiritual well-being at the forefront. It falls on us as individuals to look into these subjects and create change. We have all heard the old adage "Change starts with one." Our actions can create a ripple effect and eventually lead us to building a spiritual culture.

We will be introducing you to the philosophy of yoga as it is reflected in our eating choices. All of the recipes in this book have been designed according to the concept of ahimsa, or nonharm, which is part of the first limb of the Eight Limb Path. With ahimsa in mind, we try to cause the least harm possible to all living creatures. This is an extremely important part of yogic philosophy when it comes to eating—after all, the way most of us cause harm throughout our lives, consciously or not, is by way of what we put in our mouths.

Another precept included in the Eight Limb Path is *dhyana*, which translates to "devotion" or "meditation." In the yogic context, meditation means much more than just sitting in silence or chanting for a set amount of time. It refers to actually living our lives in a more spiritually conscious manner. The manner in which we eat offers a great avenue for infusing more mindfulness into our daily routine. With that in mind, we will also demonstrate how to eat differently, not just in terms of what you're eating but, as importantly, *how* you're eating.

Although the delicious plant-based diet we present in this book offers a ton of health and nutritional benefits, far more significantly, it opens the doorway to a greater understanding of the connection between body, mind, and spirit.

This book is not merely a cookbook, nor is it yet another guide to yoga poses. Instead, it is a jumping-off point for living a yoga life that feeds the soul and embraces the ancient writings and teachings upon which yoga was built within the context of the modern world.

Engage your mind in thinking of Me,
offer obeisances and worship Me.
Being completely absorbed in Me,
you will surely come to Me.
BHAGAVAD GITA AS IT IS **9:34**

ahimsa

Patanjali's Eight Limbs of Yoga consist of two main components: *yamas* (things we must abstain from in order to lead a spiritual and ethical yogic life) and *niyamas* (spiritual observances). The very first of the yamas is ahimsa, or nonharm. This principle lies at the very heart of yoga and should be applied to everything—how we treat ourselves, how we treat others, and how we treat the world around us.

Of course, it's logistically impossible to make it through life without causing any harm whatsoever. We live in a world in which we cannot escape creating some kind of pain. This world has been set up as being "perfectly imperfect." If we walk across a park, we will step on ants. If we wipe sweat off our forehead, we will kill millions of bacteria. So how do we create the least amount of harm while we are here on this earth? If we cannot escape killing and harming completely, then how do we minimize our footprint?

With this in mind, we do the best we can. The truth of the matter is that, even without consciously abiding by the Eight Limbs of Yoga, most of us innately attempt to live our lives in a way that doesn't inflict harm on others. However, one way in which even the most gentle and aware among us *do* cause harm is by eating in an unconscious manner. We don't stop to consider where our food is coming from or how it is making its way to our plate. For most of us, eating offers a prime avenue for becoming more aware of the earth and living beings around us and of alleviating some of the harm we are causing, often without even really being conscious of it!

One of the arguments we often hear about practicing ahimsa by eating a plant-based diet is, "Well, plants are living things, too, and you're harming them!" This is true. Every living being on this planet—whether it be a human or an animal or a tree—has what yogis call a *jiva-atma*, or a soul, residing within it.

However, again, the idea of ahimsa is to cause the *least* amount of harm possible. We like to explain it this way: let's think about the difference between eating a carrot and a cow, bearing in mind that, in each case, we are causing harm. When we eat a carrot, we harm the carrot. But to make a cow eligible for slaughter, she must weigh at least a thousand pounds. In order for cows to gain weight, they need to eat and metabolize food, just like humans do. Specifically, for a cow to gain one pound, she has to eat between sixteen and twenty pounds of grain. Let's stop and think about this for a moment. This means that before we can even think about eating a cow, an enormous number of plants have to be killed in order to feed her. Imagine how many *people* you could feed with that amount of grain, compared to the one pound of beef protein that it produces.

The harm doesn't stop there. It takes 2,500 gallons of water for a cow to produce one pound of beef. In other words, it takes 2.5 million gallons of water to get a single cow to one thousand pounds. And beyond that, animal agriculture is also one of the leading

causes of air and water pollution and deforestation. The amount of harm caused by these two environmental hazards is unquantifiable.

Now think about the fact that one-seventh of the world's population today is starving. One of the primary reasons is that most of the world's grains and produce are used to feed animals for slaughter. These animals add up to a much smaller amount of food than the grains and produce—it is food designated only for the people who can afford it. Perhaps you've heard the saying, "If everyone wanted to eat a meat-based diet, we would need two planet earths"?

But if everyone ate a plant-based diet, we could *feed* two planet earths. Aside from just harming the animals who go to slaughter, to produce them we are using up food and water resources that leave other humans wanting, and we are polluting the earth. That's a lot of harm for a single meal. And we're willing to bet that most of the people who pay into that vicious cycle have no desire to create any harm.

When we eat a vegan diet, we can avoid all of this harm—and without sacrificing any of the taste. We can feel good about our choices for ourselves and for the world around us. We are literally playing a role in decreasing the suffering of an entire planet, including the human beings, animals, plants, and the very earth we walk upon. Think of what an impact you can have by making different, mindful decisions about what you fuel your body with at least three times a day, every day of your life!

Eating this way has other advantages. When we eat vibrant whole foods in place of meat and dairy, our bodies start humming along in a more natural rhythm, making us feel both physically better and more spiritually connected. Eating a whole-food, plant-based diet nourishes our body in a unique and noticeable way because the food is of a higher quality and nutrient content than processed foods. The plethora of vitamins, minerals, and essential nutrients fuel our physical constitution at the highest level. In the same way as a car will run more smoothly for a longer period of time when it is provided with high-grade fuel, so too will our bodies. And just as our bodies are better nourished with the vitamins and minerals plants provide, so too are our brains, which makes us quicker and more alert. Spiritually, we become more attuned to the life and resources around us, and we experience a greater sense of gratitude and interconnection.

Victoria is a prime example of this. As daunting as the idea of giving up meat and meat-based products initially was to her, today there's no looking back. Not only does she feel stronger and more physically energized, but her entire life has shifted. She feels more aligned with and attuned to the world around her. She no longer searches for happiness in material things but, rather, turns to spiritual matters and meditation for fulfillment.

O son of Kunti, all that you do, all that you eat,
all that you offer and give away,
as well as all austerities that you may perform,
should be done as an offering unto Me.
BHAGAVAD GITA AS IT IS 9:27

Life as Meditation

Perhaps it sounds strange to equate our eating habits with spirituality and meditation. But, aside from the very real effects of knowing you are living life in a way that is creating minimal pain and a more sustainable world, when we eat mindfully, literally everything shifts. Another component of the Eight Limbs of Yoga involves offering all of our actions to our higher power. Everything in our life becomes spiritualized because it is all an offering. Our work becomes spiritual, our movement becomes spiritual, and our food becomes spiritual. Of course, this idea is not limited to the yogic tradition. If you grew up in a Christian household, you may have said grace before a meal. Or if you are Jewish, perhaps you eat certain foods that are symbolic in recognition of specific occasions. It's the same with yoga. We eat our meals mindfully, aware of what we have been given, and as an offering.

This doesn't have to involve more than taking a moment before we eat to ask God to accept our food or to have it first. You'll notice there's a slight difference between this and the concept of grace, wherein we thank God for being a provider. Instead, we are offering our food as if the sacred is our friend whom we want to share it with. This practice has been performed throughout the ages in India, the seat of yoga.

When Tamal explains this point to his students or workshop attendees, he often offers the following anecdote as an analogy. Every year on Tamal's birthday, our son, Kanai, asks Tamal for ten dollars. Kanai takes the ten dollars and goes to a toy store, where he buys something like Legos or a GI Joe. He then comes home and wraps the toy up in paper and duct tape. One of Tamal's favorite moments of every year is when Kanai steps into the room, gift in hand and a huge smile on his face, holding the package out for Tamal to open. Of course, Tamal doesn't need whatever toy Kanai has selected, and it was Tamal who provided the money for Kanai to purchase the toy in the first place. It's the act of exchange and what it represents that's so meaningful.

In much the same way, the Supreme Soul doesn't need the food He provides us with. After all, He's the one who gave it to us in the first place! It's the exchange that matters, from a spiritual perspective. This concept is known as *prasadam*. When we eat with the awareness of food as an exchange between ourselves and our original source, it becomes holy food, and the act of eating it becomes infused with spiritual meaning. Every time we put food into our mouths, we are building a state of awareness about our relationship with a higher power and the exchange that is constantly happening between us. Rather than just consuming, we are receiving. When we begin to look at life through this lens, our entire mind-set shifts.

From the moment we are born, our bodies are in a state of perpetual change, altering and aging. Throughout our life, our circumstances change, the locations we live in change, and so on. When our financial, physical, and mental circumstances alter, so do our ideas and the ways we perceive the world. Likewise, the more we spiritually infuse our life through acts and rituals like offering our food to the Supreme Soul, the more conscious of that which is greater than us we become aware of. We begin to adjust our mind-set into one of seeing, feeling, and willing in the direction of the spiritual.

. . . .

Feel Good, Do Good

We're sure you've heard the phrase "Food is medicine." Well, it is. And there's no doubt that when we put good things into our body, it also becomes much easier to put good stuff back out into the world. Think about your own life: we're willing to bet that when you feel sluggish and depressed, it takes extra energy to interact with those around you in a mindful, compassionate way. But when you're feeling energized and vibrant, that's what you reflect back out to those in your life and to the world in general, right?

The plant-based foods around us offer all of the minerals and nutrients we need to run like a well-oiled machine. Not only that, but they also provide us with a source of natural medicine to remedy the ailments that arise throughout the course of a life. The better you eat, the better you'll feel, and you'll learn what your body requires to run at its optimal level. The recipes included in this book will provide you with exactly the foods you need to feel good. Once you've experienced life in this bright, vitality-filled way, it's pretty hard to look back.

The recipes in this book will satisfy and excite adults, but kids will love them, too. This is great news for parents. As you begin to learn that eating mindfully is both delicious and health enhancing, you can ingrain this lifestyle in your kids so that they don't have to reprogram their thoughts about food at some point down the road. Instead, they'll grow up with the understanding that food can be used in a way that makes us feel good. Case in point: Our nine-year-old son, Kanai, has been drinking green drinks and eating salads and whole grains since he was very young. As we fed him different things, we would explain specifically how they made him strong and healthy. Because, as we know, kids are like little sponges, Kanai already knows more about food and nutrition than many adults do. He's already made the correlation on his own about how certain foods can make you feel bad or sick. When Kanai does get sick, he has an innate understanding of what foods will make him feel better and can articulate why he needs to eat a specific food or food type.

Amazingly, because Kanai has been brought up this way, he actually makes the decision to turn down cakes and sweets at birthday parties and go for healthier options because, as he puts it, "It's not good for me." (Let's be honest, this kid has some incredible willpower,

too!) We also use Kanai as an example here because he proves a big point that applies to adults and kids alike: when our baseline is to feel good, we want to keep feeling that way and are motivated to eat in a way that bolsters our health. And as our bodies begin to align themselves with natural food sources, we develop a certain rhythm that allows us to know what we need and when we need it. We are more thoughtful about our food choices, and the increased wellness that results allows us to interact with the world in a more present and energized way.

We have seen this time and time again through the myriad students that have come out of Tamal's yoga teacher training programs. Many of these students have permanently adopted a whole-food, plant-based yoga diet. These graduates constantly tell us how their lives have changed forever due to the immense amount of energy, peace, and satisfaction they have achieved by adopting a yogic diet.

life as a moving meditation

For one who sees Me everywhere and sees everything in Me,
I am never lost, nor is he ever lost to Me.
BHAGAVAD GITA AS IT IS 6:30

Most people think of meditation as a set timeframe during which we sit in silence with our eyes closed in an attempt to stop our thoughts. This is a misunderstanding of what meditation was originally designed to be. When we sit silently, it's referred to as *dharana*, or mental concentration, which is used as a premeditation exercise.

The word *meditation* actually means fixing our mind and senses on something. There is a difference between meditating on mundane matters and meditating on spiritual matters. In spiritual meditation, we fix our mind and senses on the Supreme Soul, whereas in mundane meditation, we fix our senses and mind on material things.

When we think of meditation in this way, it's easy to see how we're actually meditating all day long, whether it's on work, family, food, sex, or even social media. But there's more to it than that. We meditate when we offer our tasks at hand to God while also fixing our mind and senses on the Supreme Soul for whom we are doing it. In essence, we are consciously living our lives side by side with our original source when we maintain a mind-set that the Supreme Soul resides in our hearts.

This idea of life as a moving meditation is set forth in the Yoga Sutras. At its heart, yoga is about transforming all of our daily activities into spiritual practices so that our entire life becomes one long meditation. Believe it or not, everything from eating to working to praying to reading can be transformed into something transcendental. As you begin to incorporate this meditative mind-set into your life, the practice will become more and more natural—habitual, even. To get you started, here are some practices—or rituals, as we call them—that will set you on the path of infusing a meditative mind-set into your day-to-day life.

. . . .

Morning Rituals

MY BODY IS A TEMPLE AND A VEHICLE FOR SERVICE

The body is the material home for you, the soul, and God (*Paramatma*). Therefore, what we do with our body determines whether or not we are properly putting this material shell we have been given to good use.

We like to think of it this way: What is the difference between a bar and a temple? It totally sounds like the punch line to a joke, right? But it's not. The point here is that both a bar and a temple are made of the same materials: wood, cement, sheet rock, and nails. The only reason we treat a bar and a temple differently is because of what's inside. Now think about your body and what's residing within it: you, the soul, and the Supreme Soul. When you think about it this way, it becomes easy to treat your body as you would a temple—as a sacred place. You can use this temple to serve the original source and treat yourself better, your family better, even the entire world better.

When we wake up, standard procedure is usually to brush our teeth, groom ourselves, and head to the kitchen. When we are performing our mornings as a moving meditation, we can still do all of these things, but

A true yogi observes Me in all beings and also sees every being in Me.
Indeed the self-realized man sees Me everywhere.

BHAGAVAD GITA AS IT IS 6:29

we are simultaneously aware of our higher purpose.

Here's what we recommend. Take your time waking up; if you want, you can set your alarm clock a few minutes earlier than usual so that you don't feel pressed for time. Use this extra time to cultivate a spiritual undertone to carry with you throughout the day as you move about your life. Spend five minutes reminding yourself that you are a spiritual being having a material experience. Set your intention to use your body today to help your family, your friends, and everyone else around you get closer to the Supreme Soul.

Begin going about your morning as you normally would. Only now, because you have cultivated this mind-set, as you perform mundane tasks like brushing your teeth and taking a shower, you will do them with the mind-set of cleansing your temple. If we keep the mind-set that this body is a house for God and the soul, then we can offer our grooming, cleansing, and everything else we do to manicure our temple as an offering. It's the mind-set of knowing we are cleaning our temple that makes these actions into spiritual acts.

Everything in life is about our intentions; it's our motives that make any action self-centered or selfless, material or spiritual. For example, someone could be feeding the poor to get famous, intending to feed the hungry only until they get to a certain point of notoriety. Or someone could be feeding the poor only for the good of the people, not looking for any recognition or fame. From afar it would appear both people are doing exactly the same thing; however, the intentions are different.

This simple but powerful practice creates an entirely different outlook for you to take into your day. You'll be amazed to see how these few extra minutes in your morning carry you through any struggles and challenges that may arise, simply because you'll view them through a different lens and with a new attitude.

. . . .

Food Rituals

I OFFER THIS BACK
At any given moment, millions of people around the world are thanking God for providing them with the meal set before them. This is a great practice—but it's not yoga. In yoga, rather than looking at the Supreme Soul as a provider, we are establishing

a personal connection between ourselves and our original source.

The Yoga Sutras instruct us to offer our food back to the Supreme Soul, asking Him to accept it first. This might seem a bit strange if you are used to a more Western version of grace. If so, stop for a second and think about how you interact with friends and family at mealtimes. If someone visits your house, for instance, our guess is that, in the interest of being a good host, one of the first things you'll do is offer your guest some food or a drink. Likewise, if you are eating and your friend sits down next to you, you would probably ask them if they wanted a bite of your meal. We might not think about it, since it's such a habitual behavior, but common sense tells us that when we are in the presence of another person, we want to share some of what we have. Why should it be any different with our higher power? After all, it's that source which is providing everything in the first place, right?

The Supreme Soul doesn't need anything from us. However, offering our food up to Him is an exchange of love. And that's what's important about this ritual. In the yogic system, we strive for a constant interchange of love between ourselves and our highest source. All this takes is a simple offering in a moment of silence every time you sit down to eat, inviting the original source to have it first, just as you would with any other friend or loved one. In our house we take a pause before meals to be quiet, and with all our heart we ask the Supreme Soul, "Will you please accept this first?" Then the food is offered and considered prasadam, which means "God's mercy." The food becomes holy or spiritually purifying, and then the act of eating becomes a spiritual activity. It's like eating mantras: it cleanses our hearts and minds and brings us closer to God.

Mantras are a profound way of purifying your consciousness and connecting with the Supreme Soul. In yoga they say, "God is His name." The word *man* means "mind," and *tra* means "that which frees you from." So *mantra* means "that which frees you from your mind." We chant mantras every day as a family in our daily *kirtans* (call and response singing of mantras) and individually with our *japa* practice (repetition of God's names on mala beads), as well as when we offer our food. In reality we use mantras whenever we can. It is a nice excuse to alter our consciousness and lift up our hearts to the Supreme Soul. Whenever we drink water we think of the Bhagavad Gita, in which God says, "I am the taste of water." Then we offer the water by saying one of God's names three times: "Sri Vishnu, Sri Vishnu, Sri Vishnu."

O son of Kunti, I am the taste of water,
the light of the sun and the moon,
the syllable Om in the Vedic mantras;
I am the sound of ether and the ability in man.
BHAGAVAD GITA AS IT IS 7:8

. . . .

Rituals for Physical Movement

I AM BUILDING A STRONG TEMPLE TO CONTRIBUTE TO THE WORLD
In Western culture, fitness has become more than just a way to keep our body functioning well; it has been glamorized to sell sex. This is true of yoga in the United States as well. The practice of physical asana has become so far removed from its roots and place in traditional yoga that most practitioners are totally unaware its ultimate goal is to connect body, mind, and soul to the Supreme Soul. Today, it's much more about getting a yoga butt or dressing in the latest yoga fashion than a modality to move us closer to discovering the meaning of life.

To bring yourself back to the original intention of yoga, start your physical practice with a little prayer or by offering your practice to the Supreme Soul with the understanding that your body is being used for service and that your practice will keep that body healthy for service. This intention doesn't just apply to your asana practice; you can also perform a similar ritual of offering before jogging, swimming, or working out at the gym. Remember, yoga isn't confined to holding certain postures—it's really about a state of mind. And when we move our bodies while we are in this state of consciousness, our exercise becomes spiritualized.

Working for Love

MY WORK IS INFUSED WITH LOVE AND PURPOSE

Let's face it: every job can be a drag sometimes, but that doesn't mean your job has to be a chore day in and day out. Most of the time when we experience dissatisfaction with our job, it's because we're dreaming of doing something else or believe the grass is greener on the other side. We might fall under the misconception that if only we had another job, everything else would be better too—we'd have a better house, a nicer car, more expensive clothes, a better *life*.

What we forget is that all of those things are just temporary. There is nothing material we can acquire in this life that we will take with us when we go. It all stays here. So what *do* we take? What things are permanent? Yoga teaches us that spiritual wealth is the only possession the soul can carry with it and keep forever. Of course we need to keep our family and ourselves fed and the bills paid, but there's another frame through which we can look at our work that makes it more meaningful.

Every time you feel yourself being dragged down by work, remind yourself of its greater purpose. This job is providing you with the means to raise a spiritual family or, alternatively, to facilitate a spiritual life for yourself. You can use that job as a foundation for the care and support of your family or yourself, which will enable you to better nourish spirituality.

Forget about the "toys" we put so much emphasis on in this culture. Instead, consider another purpose for your work—become rich through simple living and high thinking. Make enough to live on, meditate, and thrive. Remove this pressure to utilize work as a way to acquire more and more, and you will find that the notion of work turns into something different: the means to an end that facilitates a more rewarding spiritual lifestyle.

Prayer is not asking, it is the longing of the soul.
It is a daily admission of one's weakness.
It is better in prayer to have a heart with no words
than words without a heart.
MAHATMA GANDHI

Meditation Rituals for Everyone

THE FAMILY THAT PRAYS TOGETHER STAYS TOGETHER

Most parents will probably agree that we want our children to be not only physically healthy but also spiritually healthy. We want to encourage the growth and health of their entire being—body, mind, and soul.

To do this, it's helpful to embed little rituals into the day to remind children about the Supreme Soul, the source from which everything comes, and to make that source a part of their daily lives. For example, every day before our family leaves the house to go to work or school, we take five minutes to meditate together. Since children have short attention spans, it can be useful to practice an interactive meditation that will keep them engaged in the moment. Remember that meditation involves fixing our mind and senses onto a particular thing. The more senses we can engage, the higher the chances our mind will follow, and our ability to stay focused will amplify. This is particularly true with kids.

One option for doing this is japa meditation, which utilizes mala or prayer beads. This technique has been used for thousands of years in India. Similar practices exist in many other spiritual traditions throughout the world; for instance, Catholics use rosary beads to focus certain prayers. You can order mala beads online, find them at a local yoga or Eastern boutique, or even make your own by stringing 108 beads together.

Once you have your mala, hold a bead between two fingers, beginning with the bead closest to the "head" of the string (where the two ends tie together). As you hold the bead, recite a Sanksrit name of God or any name for God that resonates with you as a mantra, then move on to the next bead. In our family, we like to use the mantra "Ram," which is a name for God that translates to "one who gives happiness to the soul." Continue holding each bead one at a time and reciting your mantra until you have made your way around to the last bead. This should take no more than five minutes.

All of these practices in this chapter can be applied to every facet of your life. Whenever you perform a function, no matter how mundane, you can meditate and offer your task to the Supreme Soul. Be intentional, aware of the moment and His presence. Over time, you will find that meditation is not a part of your life but, rather, is inextricable from your life.

the yoga pantry

Let food be thy medicine and let medicine be thy food.

HIPPOCRATES

When it comes to going vegan—whether the motivation is yoga or something else—one of the biggest worries people have is how daunting the logistics seem. Look around the average person's pantry, and you'll find a load of animal products and processed ingredients hidden in even the most seemingly mundane items. Going vegan can feel like you you're starting from scratch. And where *do* you start, anyway? Where will you shop now? And what should you buy? Speaking of buying things, how expensive is this going to be, anyway?

Of course, as with any other dietary style, depending upon how and where you shop, eating vegan can be expensive. But it doesn't have to be. Keeping a few staple items on hand will arm you with the basic ingredients you'll need so that you can quickly make delicious meals on the spot, even in the midst of your busy life.

The recipes included in this book have been designed so that you're not spending all of your free time sourcing obscure ingredients. (Although part of the fun of eating a plant-based diet is wandering around farmers' markets, taking in all of the vibrant colors and smells.) You should be able to find pretty much everything you'll need to get your yoga pantry up and running at your grocery store of choice, a local health food store, or online. We know how hard it is to be busy working grown-ups, so we have designed this book to be approachable and useful for everyone.

Whole Grains and Flours

BROWN RICE

Our family has a brown rice obsession; on average, we eat it at least four times per week. Its nutty flavor works well with so many dishes that it never gets old. This heart-healthy grain is low in calories, high in fiber, gluten free, and filled with a plethora of vitamins and minerals, including magnesium and manganese, which help our bodies digest fats. Because of the fiber in brown rice, it is considered a slow-release carbohydrate, which helps you maintain your blood sugar levels and keep your energy steady all day long. Not only that, but did you know that a single cup of brown rice packs in five grams of protein? Not too shabby! We cannot rave about it enough!

QUINOA

In the Dodge household, our love of brown rice is second only to our love of quinoa. In fact, we tend to alternate between the two from one day to the next, although sometimes quinoa wins out for the sole reason that it has such a short cooking time. Quinoa is gluten free, high in fiber, low in cholesterol and sodium, and a complete protein. Get this: just one quarter-cup serving fulfills 48 percent of our daily magnesium needs and has thirteen grams of protein. It is also a great source of iron.

OATS AND OAT FLOUR

High in fiber and low in fat, this lovely grain is a star. Many of our family's mornings begin with a pot of nutritious Superfood Oatmeal (page 64), accompanied with chia seeds, coconut oil, nut butters, and fresh fruit. Oats are packed with vitamins and minerals, including manganese, phosphorus, magnesium, selenium, zinc, and copper. Oat groats are the original whole form oats are harvested in, but most people prefer rolled, crushed, or steel-cut oats. Oat flour is incredibly easy to make at home and is great for using in baked goods. Make sure to buy gluten-free oats if you have any gluten allergies or sensitivities.

BUCKWHEAT

Technically not a grain, buckwheat is a seed that is high in both fiber and protein. Since it often serves the purpose of a grain in cooking, we're taking a bit of creative license here. Buckwheat is a complete protein, containing all nine essential amino acids. To maximize its nutritional content, we use it in its raw form, called buckwheat groats, as opposed to its roasted form, called kasha. Raw buckwheat is gluten free and simple to make into flour for baking.

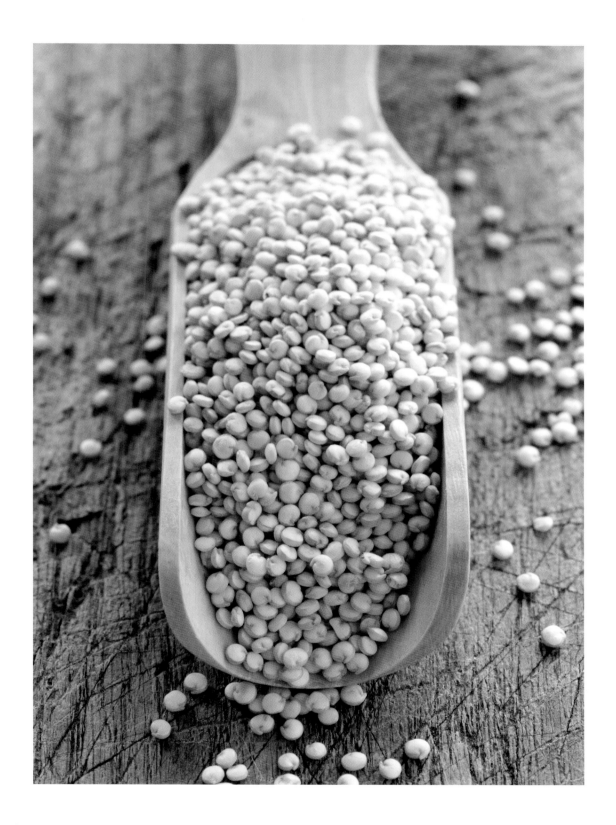

100 PERCENT WHITE WHOLE-WHEAT PASTRY FLOUR

White whole-wheat pastry flour is a great replacement for all-purpose flour (aka white flour) in baking because it is light in texture, as opposed to whole-wheat flour, which is very dense. It does contain gluten, so if you're gluten intolerant, white whole-wheat pastry flour isn't for you. We like Bob's Red Mill organic whole-wheat pastry flour or King Arthur brand, which can be purchased at health food stores or online.

SPELT FLOUR

Spelt is an ancient grain that has a nutty and slightly sweet flavor. When baking, we often swap out white whole-wheat pastry flour for spelt flour because the spelt version isn't cross-pollinated with other grains like wheat is. It is also richer than wheat in nutrients, such as protein and minerals. It does contain gluten, so if you have a gluten allergy or sensitivity be sure to use an alternative flour, such as garbanzo bean or oat flour.

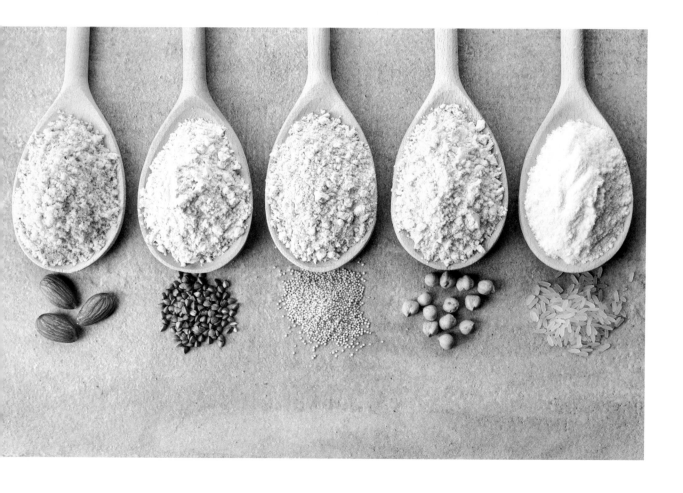

Beans and Legumes

CHICKPEAS (GARBANZOS) AND GARBANZO BEAN FLOUR

Chickpeas are one of the most popular and versatile of all legumes. They are especially popular in Indian cuisine. We love using whole chickpeas to make hummus and soups and roasted as a crunchy crouton alternative, and garbanzo bean flour is a great alternative for gluten-free diets. Tamal uses this protein-packed gluten- and grain-free flour in his delicious savory Chickpea Breakfast Crepe recipe (page 66), one of our daughter Savannah's favorite breakfast dishes. A half cup of garbanzo bean flour has about ten grams of protein.

BLACK BEANS

We always seem to have a mason jar filled with black beans soaking in water. Our son, Kanai, is obsessed with black beans and would eat them for every meal every day if he could. We fully support his obsession: black beans are loaded with nourishing things, such as protein, fiber, antioxidants, and micronutrients. They will keep you full and give you steady, consistent energy throughout the day. Black beans are great in tacos or in our Hearty Vegan Chili (page 117).

LENTILS

Lentils are a daily go-to food in our family. They are full of fiber, are easy to digest, and can be prepared in a jiffy. We throw on a pot of lentils in the morning while we're getting ready for the day and then have a staple to play with after we return from our morning meetings or workouts. We use french lentils, black lentils, green lentils, red lentils, and yellow lentils. There is so much you can make with these gems! Try our Bombay Red Lentil Soup (page 118) for a nutritious and delicious all-in-one meal.

One cup of cooked lentils has about eighteen grams of protein and fifteen grams of fiber, making them one of the most filling stick-to-your-ribs foods there is. They are also packed with minerals, such as folate, manganese, phosphorus, and iron, and are very alkalizing to the body, which is hard to find in a protein. To get even more nutritional value, you can soak and sprout them. Soaking and sprouting lentils increases their nutritional value and makes them even easier to digest. They become sweet in taste and are great for tossing on top of a salad.

AVOID CANNED BEANS

Preparing dried beans from scratch allows you to sidestep the sodium and other additives that canned beans contain. In fact, in general, we should all use fresh or frozen foods as much as possible in order to avoid cans.

Cans are often laced with the dangerous toxin bisphenol A (also known as BPA), which can leach into the foods. BPA is an artificial estrogen that has been linked with heart disease, blood sugar issues, miscarriages, low testosterone in men, and prostate and breast cancer.

Canned foods generally contain astronomical levels of sodium—up to 15 percent more than their noncanned, home-cooked counterparts. Excess sodium can cause high blood pressure and other heart issues. It is much better to prepare your own foods in order to control the amount of sodium in your diet.

Canned foods also contain sulfites, preservatives added to foods to extend their shelf life. Many people are seriously sensitive to sulfites, and others are a little less sensitive but still react. Sulfites can cause such reactions as wheezing, coughing, and skin rashes. Sulfites can also appear under the aliases sulfur dioxide, potassium bisulfite, potassium metabisulfite, and sodium sulfite.

Another problem with canned foods is that they are heated to an extreme degree for a long time. The high temperatures kill off any bacteria or pathogens that may be in the food, but this process also kills off many heat-sensitive vitamins and minerals, and it changes the structure of the proteins in the foods. The reason canned foods last so long is because anything that could degrade them has been killed!

If you are short on time, can't soak and cook your beans from scratch, or opt to use canned foods, be sure to get organic options that are in BPA-free cans.

DIY PRESERVING

It's important to soak dried beans in a large, uncovered bowl of water at room temperature for at least eight to ten hours prior to cooking. Soaking the beans not only lessens the cooking time but also improves their digestibility and increases their nutritional content. After you have finished soaking the beans, be sure to thoroughly rinse them with water to remove unwanted elements, such as the flatulence-causing substances you are trying to eliminate by soaking the beans in the first place. It's also important not to add any salt to the beans before cooking them because it will cause them to cook unevenly.

Nuts and Seeds

ALMONDS

Almonds are one of our favorite nuts. High in vitamin E, they are amazing for your skin. Almonds also are loaded with fiber, protein, magnesium, copper, and manganese. They contain a probiotic component, so they aid in digestion. We tend to use most of our almonds for our Raw Vanilla Almond Milk (page 39); however, we also eat them straight up as a snack or put them in our Farmhouse Granola (page 54).

CASHEWS

Cashews are king in our kitchen. We are obsessed with making our Cashew Cream Everything Sauce (page 198), which we drizzle on everything from tacos or salads to whole-grain bowls, and our out-of-this-world Cauliflower Mash (page 98). Creamy and rich when soaked and blended, cashews are super versatile and can be used in savory or sweet dishes, like our Raw Lemon Raspberry Cheesecake (page 216). Loaded with vitamin E, minerals such as magnesium and zinc, and rich in antioxidants, cashews are a great addition to any plant-based diet.

CHIA SEEDS

Cha-cha-cha chia! Chia seeds are so fun to cook with. These tiny black powerhouse seeds are packed with incredible nutrients, such as omega-3 fatty acids, antioxidants, calcium, magnesium, potassium, fiber, and protein. We make chia pudding almost every day and throw a spoonful of chia seeds into our Superfood Oatmeal (page 64) and smoothies. Try our Cha-Cha-Cha Chia Pudding (page 72) before a workout for a burst of energy.

FLAXSEEDS

These tiny seeds are bursting with omega-3s and fiber. The best way to absorb flaxseeds is to grind them up. We add them to our oatmeal or drop a tablespoon into our smoothies. Ground flaxseeds are also a great replacement for eggs. You can combine one tablespoon of flax meal with three tablespoons of water and let the mixture sit until it thickens, about ten minutes. As it thickens, it forms a gel-like substance that resembles an egg white. Make sure to store your flaxseeds in the refrigerator or freezer, because they tend to go rancid quickly.

If you are short on time, we have a cheat on the soaking method. We use hot water and soak the cashews for about 15–20 minutes. This works like a charm.

HEMP SEEDS

Hemp seeds—called "hemp hearts" when they're shelled—are the seeds of the hemp plant. They are an excellent source of omega-3 and omega-6, containing an ideal ratio of three to one. They are a complete protein and offer a whopping eighteen grams of protein in just one-quarter cup! Nutty in flavor, hemp seeds are a perfect salad topping, give a little oomph to our Superfood Oatmeal (page 64) and Refreshing Summer Quinoa Salad (page 143) dishes, and are a great smoothie add-in. Ground hemp protein powder is an incredible way to power up your postworkout smoothie, because it helps alkalize your body and assists in muscle recovery.

PUMPKIN SEEDS (PEPITAS)

These powerhouse seeds are loaded with protein, iron, magnesium, and zinc. Just a half cup of pumpkin seeds packs in twenty-five grams of protein. We like to use pepitas in salads or soaked overnight to be added to our morning smoothies.

. . . .

Healthy Fats

COCONUT OIL

We could write an entire book on the benefits of coconut oil (and, in fact, many people already have!). We use coconut oil every day in some way, shape, or form, from adding it to our Farmhouse Granola (page 54) to melting it in a cast-iron pan to heat up leftovers. Not only is coconut oil great as a food, but it also makes a terrific skin moisturizer and is excellent for oil pulling, an Ayurvedic practice by which you extract toxins from the body by swishing a teaspoon of oil in your mouth for ten to twenty minutes. Here is just a brief list of the many reasons coconut oil should be a staple in your pantry:

- Has antibacterial, antiviral, antiparasitic, and antifungal properties

- Is loaded with vitamin E

- Contains lauric acid, a component found in mother's milk

- Contains medium-chain fatty acids, which go directly to the liver and turn straight into energy, increasing metabolism

- Makes a great hair conditioner

- Is beneficial to your heart

- Improves your digestive system

- Strengthens your immune system

- Speeds up the healing of bruises, cuts, and infections when applied topically

OLIVE OIL

One of the healthiest oil options, olive oil contains healthy fats and is loaded with antioxidants, which enhance heart health. It has also been used for thousands of years for skin, nail, and hair hydration. Olive oil is great in recipes such as our Fresh and Creamy Pesto (page 197) or as the perfect simple topping for pasta with tomatoes and basil.

When shopping for olive oil, be sure to look specifically for cold-pressed extra-virgin olive oil, which is high in monounsaturated fatty acids and antioxidants (in other words, it's heart healthy). Olive oil should be housed in a glass bottle and stored in a dark, cool place to keep out light and prevent the oil from going rancid.

GRAPE-SEED OIL

Grape-seed oil is our go-to for sautéing veggies and roasting potatoes, like those in our Autumn Roasted Veggies recipe (page 110). Its clean, light, neutral flavor works well in baked goods as well. This oil is also amazing for high-heat cooking because, like coconut oil, its molecular structure isn't altered by high temperatures. Not only is it nourishing for your hair and skin because of its vitamin E content, but it also contains omega-6 fatty acid, which plays an important role in brain function, skin and hair growth, and metabolism regulation.

AVOCADO

Creamy, dreamy avocado. Really, what's better? We often find ourselves eating avocados straight out of their skins, with nothing more than a sprinkle of salt and pepper. As they're bursting with healthy fats, fiber, and more potassium than a banana, we seem to eat at least one or two a day. At one point, we had an avocado tree in our yard, and it felt like an endless supply of pure gold was right at our doorstep. Try it in our Creamy Chocolate Pudding (page 219) or Coconut Ceviche (page 134). In our book, this is one of *the* best fats to include in your daily diet.

Sweeteners

DATES

Dates have been used as a delicious treat and a medicinal food for thousands of years. In the Islamic faith, for the month of Ramadan, practitioners abstain from eating during the day and take only a small meal at night. When Muslims break their fast in the evening, it's with dates and water. Dates are so nutrient dense that they satisfy those who are fasting and help them ease into eating a full meal without complications once the month is up.

Dates are filled with good sugar, fiber, and minerals, such as iron, calcium, phosphorus, zinc, potassium, and magnesium. Not to mention a plethora of vitamins, like vitamin A, vitamin K, thiamin, niacin, folate, and riboflavin. We use dates in smoothies, oatmeal, baked goods, and even piecrusts—or just as a snack in their own right. Dates truly are nature's candy! They provide incredible preworkout fuel because they boost your energy and fill your muscles with glycogen, which is what your body needs to carry you though physical hurdles.

MAPLE SYRUP

Maple syrup isn't just for pancakes; it can also be used as an alternative sweetener for teas, smoothies, baked goods, and just about anything else you want to sweeten up. Maple syrup and its derivative, maple sugar, were first discovered by indigenous people in what is now called North America long before European settlers arrived. Tribes enjoyed the sweet sap as a staple in their communities and harvested and traded it amongst themselves. We use it in our Cha-Cha-Cha Chia Pudding (page 72) and scrumptious Raw Lemon Raspberry Cheesecake (page 216). All sweeteners have sucrose, but maple syrup has a bit less than cane sugar and also has many antioxidants and minerals that are very beneficial. This is a distinguishing factor, because most sweeteners have high calories but little nutritional content. And with its high levels of antioxidants, which protect cells from DNA damage, maple syrup helps fight off free radicals and inflammation.

COCONUT SUGAR

Coconut sugar is made from the sap produced by the bud stem of coconuts. This sap contains nutritional electrolytes like potassium, magnesium, and sodium. Coconut sugar also brings to the table minerals such as iron, zinc, and calcium, not to mention it is lower on the glycemic index than refined sugar. We use coconut sugar in our Vegan Banana Walnut Date Bread (page 69) and sometimes as a replacement in recipes that call for brown sugar.

· · · · ·

Salt

HIMALAYAN PINK SALT

Himalayan pink salt is pretty much the only salt we use in our house. Did you know table salt contains *zero* nutrients? What it does contain is chemicals and sugar. Sea salt contains more minerals than table salt, but not as many as Himalayan pink salt, which boasts the highest content of minerals — eighty-four, to be exact! Sprinkle it on your salad or add a pinch on top of your raw cacao smoothie. The difference in taste will astound you.

· ·

Getting Organized

PLAN YOUR MENUS

One of the biggest hurdles when it comes to staying healthy is being organized about your food purchases. Often, people go to the grocery store and just buy food impulsively, a little of this and a little of that. To get organized, plan a menu, especially if you have a family. You can make quick, easy meals on days the kids have extracurricular activities and save longer meal preparation for when you are relaxed at home. The key is to preplan the week. If you draw up a menu, it will make your shopping trip smooth and easy. Write a detailed shopping list and then break it into categories according to your store's layout. You will see that you end up spending less money, since you will buy only what you need.

You will not be impulsive, or at least not to the extent you might have been without a planned-ahead menu.

ORGANIZE YOUR SHOPPING

Here are a few simple tips.

1 Choose foods that you can use more than once in a week, such as brown rice and salad greens.

2 Try to shop at your local farmers' market for produce and always try to buy seasonally. The produce will taste better if it is in season and not preharvested and flown in from distant locations. If you can't get to a farmers' market, don't worry. Shop for in-season, organic produce at your local grocery store.

3 If you can, designate one day a week "shopping day." For instance, we shop on Saturday morning. That is when our farmers' market is open, so we go there first and then to Trader Joe's or our local grocery store to do the rest of our shopping.

4 Organize your food as soon as you get home. Basically, try to categorize the foods you buy into groups so ingredients are easy to find when you are making a recipe. See "Organize Your Kitchen" below for some simple guidelines.

READ LABELS

Learn how to read food labels. More often than not, what you cannot pronounce is not healthy for your body. A good rule of thumb is: *The fewer ingredients the better.* When something is whole wheat, it should be labeled "whole wheat," not just "wheat." If you see "wheat flour," it means refined white flour. Similarly, for rice, the label should state "whole-grain brown rice" or "brown rice." If it states only "rice," this means it is refined white rice.

Sugars are secretly hidden within other names, and you have to be a bit of a detective to find them. Just to list a few of the names you should avoid: sucrose, corn syrup, high-fructose corn syrup, dextrose, fructose, corn sweetener.

Also, ingredients are listed in descending order by weight, so the position of the ingredient can give you an idea if there is a lot or just a smidge in the package. It takes practice to understand labels, so be patient. Bring a pen and paper and write things down while you are shopping if you don't know what they are. Then go home and look them up. It feels great to educate yourself, especially when it comes to what you put in your precious body.

ORGANIZE YOUR KITCHEN

Beyond preplanning your meals, you can make maintaining a healthy lifestyle easier if you take the time to organize your entire kitchen. It will function so much more smoothly if everything has its place. Even if you have a small kitchen, you can do this. Clean your veggies as soon as you get home from shopping and store them in containers so that you can access them easily. Put all of your grains, dried beans, and legumes in one place, breads and pastas in another, baking ingredients in another. Potatoes and onions go together. Spices. Fruit. Even the freezer should be organized, with frozen fruit in one section and frozen veggies in another section. Use the top of the refrigerator for storage if necessary. We do. Keep oils together in a dark, cool cupboard. We store nuts and seeds in the refrigerator or the freezer, since they can go rancid fast. Keep your refrigerator clean. Make sure you can see everything easily. You can even push for extreme organization and label containers. We did that at one point, but we buy too much of a variety of foods to continually keep track. You could try making generic labels that fit multiple ingredients, like "greens" instead of "spinach." That would work well.

GET STARTED!

Go into your kitchen and think about where you need to clean up and reorganize. Give it a deep clean to get started. Throw away anything that is not going to serve your body moving forward. Processed foods, bad oils, refined sugars—toss them. I know it will be hard. No one likes to waste food, but these foods will just deplete your body and make you toxic. Let's look forward to a beautiful, new, glowing you! Feed your family a rainbow of succulent fruits and veggies. Start using whole grains instead of refined, meaning brown instead of white. Choose coconut oil and olive oil and toss out the canola and vegetable oils. Buy fresh herbs! In the next chapter you will learn how to create dishes with these natural ingredients that God gave us in their organic, pure state.

OUR FAVORITE KITCHEN TOOLS AND EQUIPMENT

The food for a plant-based lifestyle can be quite simple to prepare. It's important, though, to have the right tools. There are some kitchen tools and appliances that we just can't live without. Well, we actually could if we really had to, but we use them on a daily basis. Here are our top three: a good blender, a food processor, and a very sharp knife! We've listed our favorite brands and utensils, including those top three, below.

Blender

This is the one piece of equipment we use on a daily basis. We pretty much make one smoothie a day. We use a Blendtec. However, the Vitamix is right up there in quality and power, so either one receives a thumbs-up from us. A good blender is a bit of an investment, but you will never regret spending the money, once you realize how useful and reliable it is. It'll last for years!

Food Processor

We have a fourteen-cup Cuisinart food processor that we love. We use it for just about everything, from pesto and hummus to nut butters, desserts, and more. If you are just starting out on this plant-based food journey, the fourteen-cup food processor is not necessarily what you need. We recommend beginning with a seven- or ten-cup version, which should suit your needs. We also have the mini (four-cup) processor and use it for dressings and sauces. The four-cup version works wonders when you need to chop up garlic and onions.

Chef's Knife

If you have only one good, sharp knife, that is all you will need. We have tried all kinds of knives, and our favorites are J. A. Henckels and MAC knives. They are the sharpest and easiest to handle. We have tried ceramic knives. They're great tools, but they always end up chipping.

Cast-Iron Skillet

A cast-iron skillet is essential in our kitchen. We use these durable pans for a few different reasons. They distribute heat evenly. They release trace amounts of iron into your food, helping you get part of your daily dose. And once you season them, they are naturally nonstick pans. A win-win for us!

Citrus Juicer

You can buy an expensive juicer, and we have in the past. However, we've also come to realize that a simple hand juicer works well, particularly if you are juicing lemons, limes, and oranges. One, it's easier to clean, and two, it's more space efficient. In time, you'll start to run out of room to store all your kitchen contraptions. Trust us, we have our share! Sometimes simple is better.

Nut Milk Bags

We use these bags to make our Raw Vanilla Almond Milk (page 39) about twice a week. The bags are easy to find on Amazon. We use the 12x12 reusable kind.

Mason Jars

We have so many mason jars in so many shapes and sizes, it's comical. We use them for storing soups, sauces, and nut milks. We use the extra-large ones in our pantry for storing beans and grains. They also make great containers for gifts. During the holidays, Victoria makes her Farmhouse Granola (page 54) with cranberries instead of raisins and hands it out as gifts to teachers, coaches, friends, and family. These beauties are a must in our kitchen.

Spiralizer

We mostly use this gadget for our zucchini noodles, but there is much more you can do with a spiralizer. It is inexpensive and so much fun. The kids will want to get involved in mealtime with a tool like this. You can simply go to Amazon to get a basic version, which will cost you about thirty dollars. It makes a great gift for chef friends, too!

Extra-Large Baking Sheets and Parchment Paper

We love to bake, and when we do, we like to employ the large baking sheets (12x17) for big batches of roasted veggies, potatoes, black bean burgers, and, of course, cookies and granola. These are multipurpose and get plenty of use in our house. We line them with unbleached parchment paper for a quick cleanup.

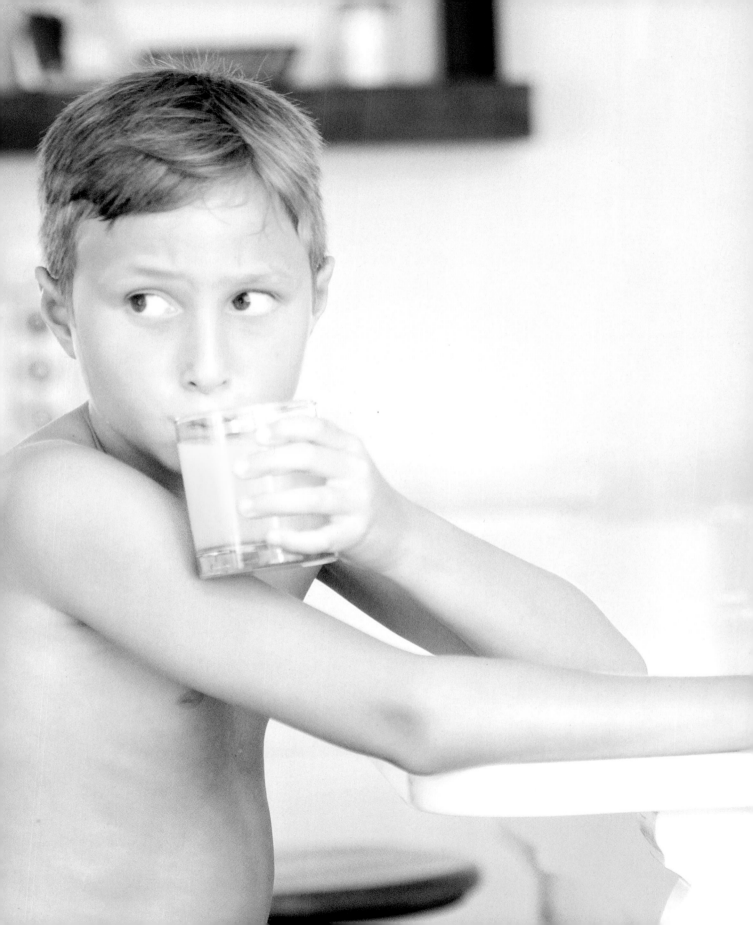

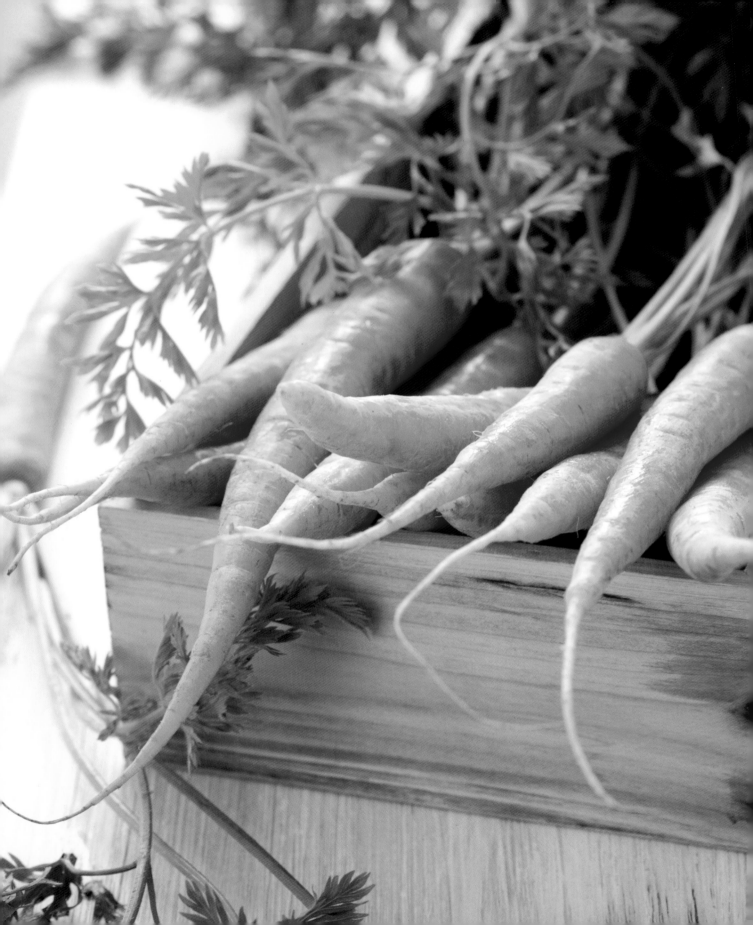

the recipes

The food you eat can be either the safest and most powerful form
of medicine or the slowest form of poison.

ANN WIGMORE

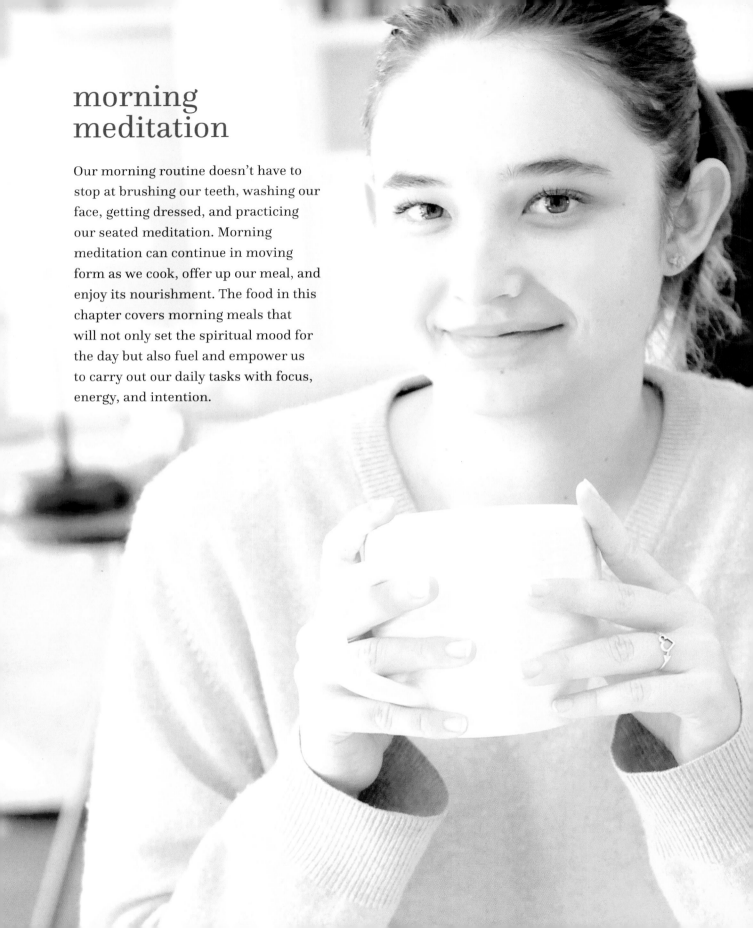

morning meditation

Our morning routine doesn't have to stop at brushing our teeth, washing our face, getting dressed, and practicing our seated meditation. Morning meditation can continue in moving form as we cook, offer up our meal, and enjoy its nourishment. The food in this chapter covers morning meals that will not only set the spiritual mood for the day but also fuel and empower us to carry out our daily tasks with focus, energy, and intention.

smoothies and teas

Chocolate–Peanut Butter Smoothie

SERVES 2

Chocolate and peanut butter are the ultimate power couple. Sweet, creamy chocolate plus salty peanut butter, and then a banana to bring it all together . . . it won't last long in the glass! And it's so full of nutrition, you won't mind pouring a second helping. This smoothie delivers healthy fats, potassium, fiber, and loads of antioxidants. How often can you drink something that tastes like dessert and feel good about it?

1 cup unsweetened
almond milk

½ cup water

1 frozen banana

2 Tbsp. peanut butter
or almond butter

1 Tbsp. raw cacao powder

½ cup ice

1 scoop vegan vanilla protein
powder, 1–2 pitted dates
(preferably Medjool), or 1
tsp. maple syrup (optional)

1 Place all ingredients into a high-powered blender and blend until smooth. Add a little more water if you'd like it less thick.

2 If you are not using a vegan protein powder, you can blend in the dates or maple syrup to give it a little more sweetness.

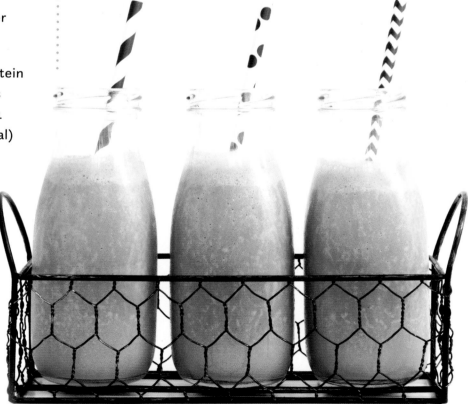

Raw Vanilla Almond Milk

MAKES ABOUT 3 CUPS

"Milk: it does a body good" is a slogan many of us grew up with in Western culture. This Raw Vanilla Almond Milk fulfills that promise. It's creamy, sweet, smooth, and full of goodness. Store-bought nut milks are often loaded with toxic fillers and sweeteners, but this almond milk is clean and pure. Once you've tried it, you will never want to drink any other kind of nut milk again. It is seriously addicting!

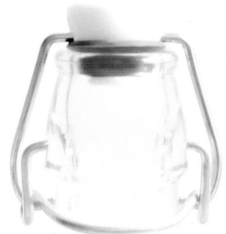

1 cup raw almonds, soaked for 6–8 hours

3 cups water

⅛ tsp. vanilla bean powder or ½ tsp. vanilla extract

⅛ tsp. Himalayan pink salt

1 Tbsp. maple syrup

. . . .

1 Place all ingredients in a high-powered blender and blitz for 45 seconds, or until smooth.

2 Over a medium-size bowl, pour the almond mixture into a cheesecloth or nut milk bag. Squeeze the mixture through the cheesecloth or bag until you get as much of the milk out as possible.

3 Pour the milk into a glass milk bottle or container and refrigerate for at least 2 hours before serving. The almond milk will last for up to 5 days.

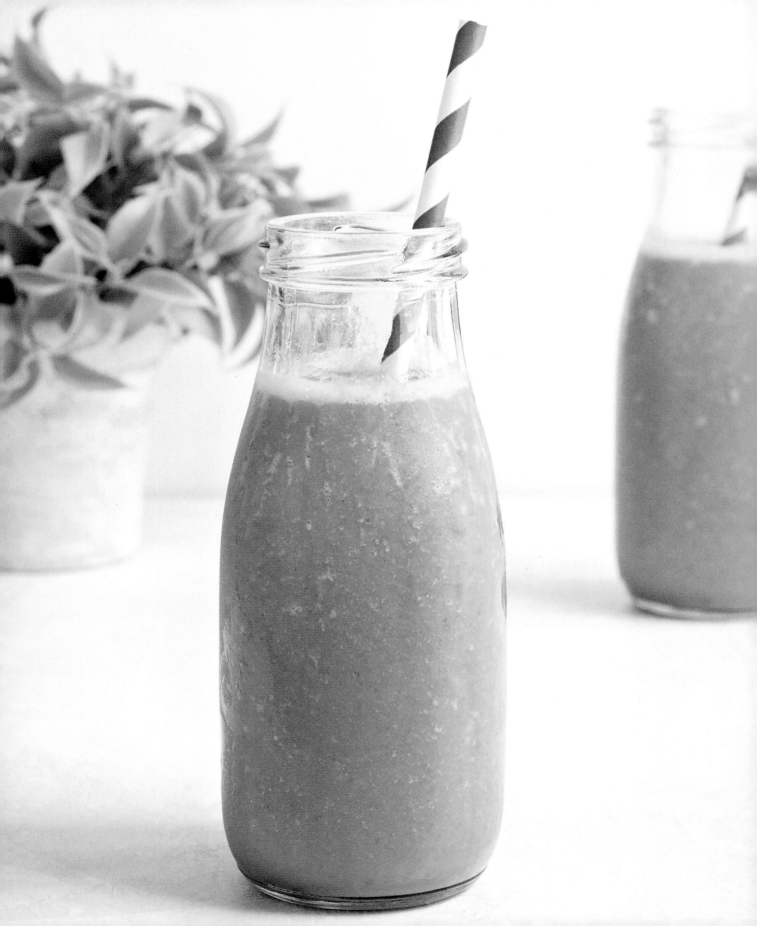

The Yogi

It's not always easy to squeeze in your daily dose of greens, but you can start your day off right by throwing those leafy veggies into your smoothie first thing in the morning. That way, you know you got at least one serving in. The Yogi offers that perfect start to set the pace and help you make healthier choices throughout the day. It is filled with wholesome nutrients, like fiber, calcium, potassium, vitamin E, and vitamin C. It's also a great drink to enjoy one hour before or after yoga class, to replenish those nutrients in your body.

1 cup unsweetened almond milk

1 cup organic spinach or kale

½ cup water

½ cup frozen pineapple chunks

1 celery stalk

1 frozen banana

½ organic Fuji apple, seeded and chopped

2 pitted dates (preferably Medjool)

2–3 ice cubes

1 In a high-speed blender, combine all of the ingredients and blend until smooth. Pour into glasses and enjoy!

You can add 1 Tbsp. of vegan protein powder to make a great postworkout recovery smoothie.

Blueberry Beauty

SERVES 2

Who doesn't love blueberries? They are so beautiful and vibrant in color. Loaded with antioxidants and fiber, these little gems are powerhouses. They are low on the glycemic scale and contain heaps of potassium, folate, vitamin C, and vitamin B6. The nutritional benefits also include healthy fats and omegas, protein, and vitamin E. This smoothie is bursting with so many subtle flavors your tongue will dance with joy!

1 cup fresh or frozen blueberries

1 cup unsweetened almond milk

2 pitted dates (preferably Medjool)

1 Tbsp. coconut oil

1 Tbsp. almond butter

1 Tbsp. hemp seeds

½ tsp. vanilla extract

¼ tsp. cinnamon

4–5 ice cubes

1–2 Tbsp. water (optional)

Toppings of choice (optional)

1   Place all the ingredients into a high-speed blender and blend until smooth. Add 1–2 Tbsp. of water if you would like the smoothie to be a little thinner.

2   Garnish with a few more hemp seeds, a sprinkle of cinnamon or other toppings before serving.

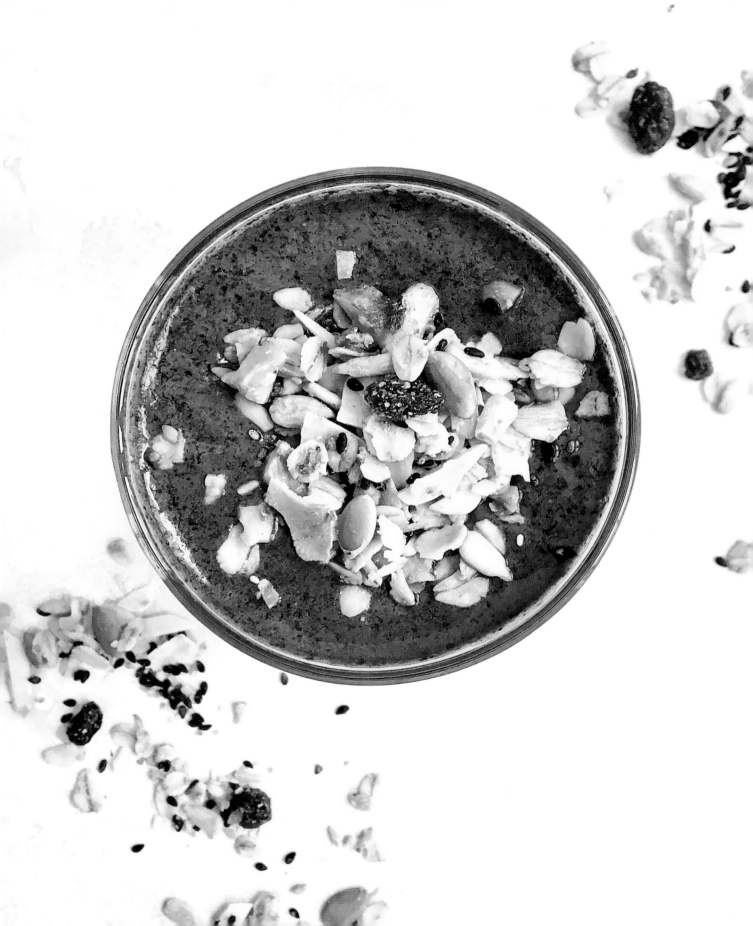

On-the-Go Hemp and Almond Butter Smoothie

SERVES 2

With more than 18 grams of plant protein, this smoothie packs a lot of goodness into just one glass. Bursting with fiber, potassium, and omegas, too, it is is a perfect breakfast for the busy parent, athlete, or business owner. It's good to mix up your plant proteins, so we often throw this into our smoothie lineup. Nom-nom.

1 cup unsweetened almond milk

1 frozen banana

1 cup spinach

2 Tbsp. almond butter

2 Tbsp. hemp protein powder

2 pitted dates (preferably Medjool)

¼ cup water

4–5 ice cubes (optional)

1 Place all ingredients in a high-speed blender and blend until smooth. Serve immediately.

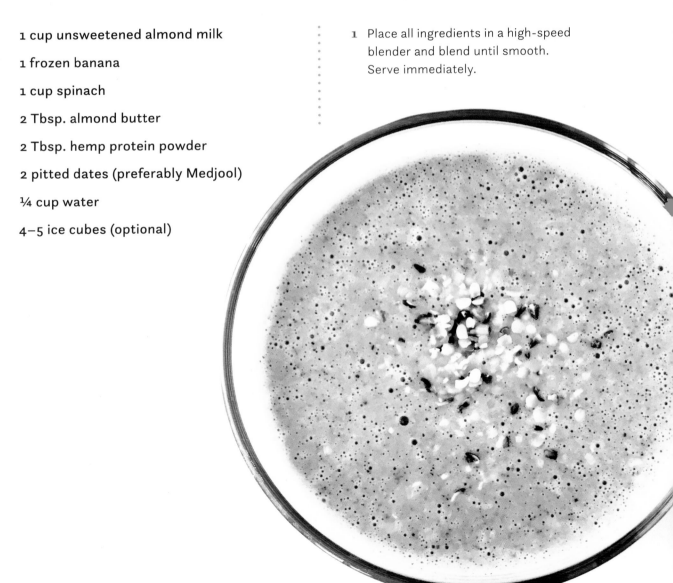

Pretty in Pink Pitaya Smoothie

SERVES 2

This drink is so pretty, it's like a pink sunrise in a glass. It's also loaded with amazing nutrients. The pitaya is low in calories, high in fiber, and full of antioxidants, magnesium, and vitamin C. And the almond butter and almond milk are packed with vitamin E. It's the perfect drink not just to enjoy but also to boost your immune system. And don't forget that color—the most beautiful pink on the planet.

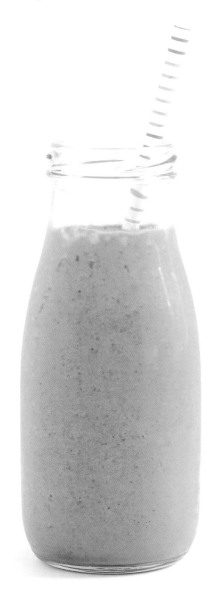

1 cup unsweetened almond or coconut milk

1 3.5-oz. packet frozen pitaya or 1 cup fresh pitaya

1 cup frozen raspberries

½ frozen banana

1 heaping Tbsp. almond butter

2–3 pitted dates (preferably Medjool)

½ cup water

1 scoop plant-based protein powder (optional)

1 Blend all ingredients in a high-powered blender until smooth and creamy. If you want a thinner consistency, add a bit more water.

To make this into a smoothie bowl, omit the water and use a whole frozen banana instead.

Banana Cinnamon Bliss

SERVES 2

The title says it all. It is a glass full of bliss! This creamy banana cinnamon smoothie is a perfect preworkout drink. The dates will give you a great energy boost, while the fat in the almond butter will slowly release the sugars from the banana. This smoothie is on the lighter side but is bursting with healthy nutrients, like potassium, fiber, magnesium, and calcium. The almond milk is rich in vitamins and minerals, especially vitamin E. Cinnamon is loaded with antioxidants, too. So whether you are about to work out or not, pour yourself a glass to start your day!

1 cup unsweetened almond milk

⅓ cup water

1 frozen banana

1 Tbsp. almond butter

2 pitted dates (preferably Medjool)

½ tsp. vanilla extract

¼ tsp. cinnamon

Pinch of Himalayan pink salt

4 ice cubes

1. Place ingredients in a high-speed blender and blend until smooth.

Try adding a little cardamom to vary the taste.

Piña Colada Summer Smoothie

Take yourself to the beach with this refreshing, revitalizing tropical smoothie. With every sip, you'll be transported to an idyllic getaway with white sands and crystal-blue waters—it's that good! It's best suited for a warm summer day, but it can also serve as a fun pick-me-up during the winter months. This smoothie is filled with healthy nutrients, coconut milk fats, enzymes, potassium, vitamin C, and fiber. Make a double batch and treat the whole neighborhood to a holiday in a glass. (Well, that's what happens at our house.) You can also freeze this smoothie into yummy popsicles.

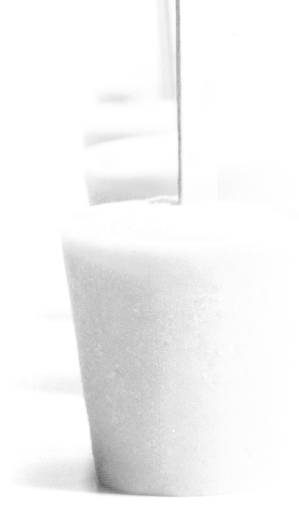

1½ cups coconut milk

1½ cups frozen pineapple chunks

1 frozen banana

½ cup frozen mango chunks

2 Tbsp. maple syrup

2 tsp. vanilla extract

4 ice cubes

1 Place all ingredients in a blender and process on high speed until you have a creamy, smooth consistency.

Watermelon Coconut Mint Cooler

SERVES 4

This mouthwatering, hydrating Watermelon Coconut Mint Cooler will satisfy your every craving during the hottest months of the year. We love to use the coconut water from fresh young Thai coconuts, which have the sweetest and best taste. It takes more work to get the coconut water from these than from other varieties, but it is well worth it. Wait until you taste all of the flavors of the heavenly ingredients in this lip-smacking cooler—it's one more reason to hope that summer will last just a bit longer!

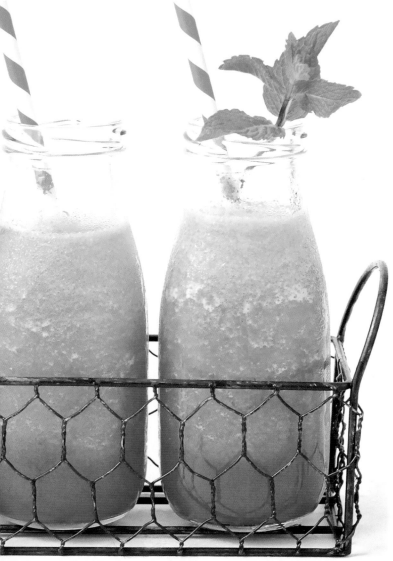

1 small watermelon

16 oz. coconut water (preferably from young Thai coconuts)

Handful of fresh mint leaves

Juice from 1 lime

1 Cut open, seed, and cube the fresh watermelon. You should have about 6 cups of watermelon cubes. Discard the seeds and freeze the cubes overnight.

2 Place the frozen watermelon cubes, coconut water, mint leaves, and lime juice in a blender. Blend at high speed until the mixture looks like a slushie.

If your kids would like this drink to be a little sweeter, you can blend in 1 Tbsp. of maple syrup or your choice of sweetener.

Hemp Matcha Latte

SERVES 1

First thing in the morning, there's nothing like holding a mug filled with a warm, delicious, and nourishing drink in your hands. This Hemp Matcha Latte contains 10 grams of protein and heaps of antioxidants. So you can enjoy a cozy tea and feel energized all at once. Victoria doesn't drink caffeine, so you can follow her lead and go as light on the matcha as you want. A good-quality matcha is bright green and smooth. It will not taste bitter at all; there will be a slightly sweet taste. We like ceremonial-grade matcha. Here's to your health!

8 oz. hot water

2 Tbsp. hemp seeds

2 Tbsp. maple syrup

¼ tsp. powdered matcha green tea

1   In a high-powered blender, pour the hot water, hemp seeds, maple syrup, and powdered matcha. Blend until smooth and creamy. Serve immediately.

When blending hot liquids, use caution to avoid potentially dangerous pressure building up in your blender or food processor. Good safety techniques include blending in smaller batches, pausing every so often to lift the lid and release the steam, or using an immersion blender instead of a countertop blender.

Kanai's Peanut Butter and Jelly Smoothie

SERVES 2

Let your kids explore and play in the kitchen. Trust us! You'll be surprised and delighted with the dishes they come up with. In the process, they'll learn about health and whole, nourishing foods. This will set them up for later in life, when they're taking care of themselves and their own families. When we set our son, Kanai, free in the kitchen, he conjured up this Peanut Butter and Jelly Smoothie. Then we helped him refine the recipe. This is a sweet and naturally delicious drink, a treat for children and grown-ups alike.

1 cup unsweetened almond milk

1 cup frozen grapes

½ cup frozen strawberries

1 giant spoonful of peanut butter
(we use about 2 Tbsp.)

1   Place all ingredients in a high-speed blender and blend until smooth and creamy.

Frozen grapes are a perfect after-school snack, party appetizer, or late-night treat.

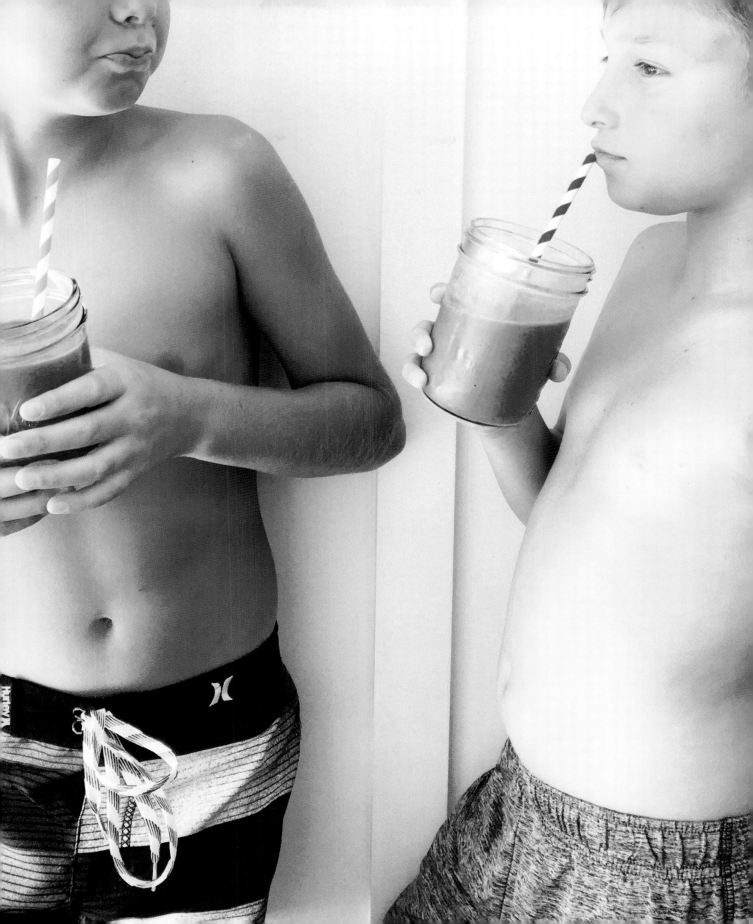

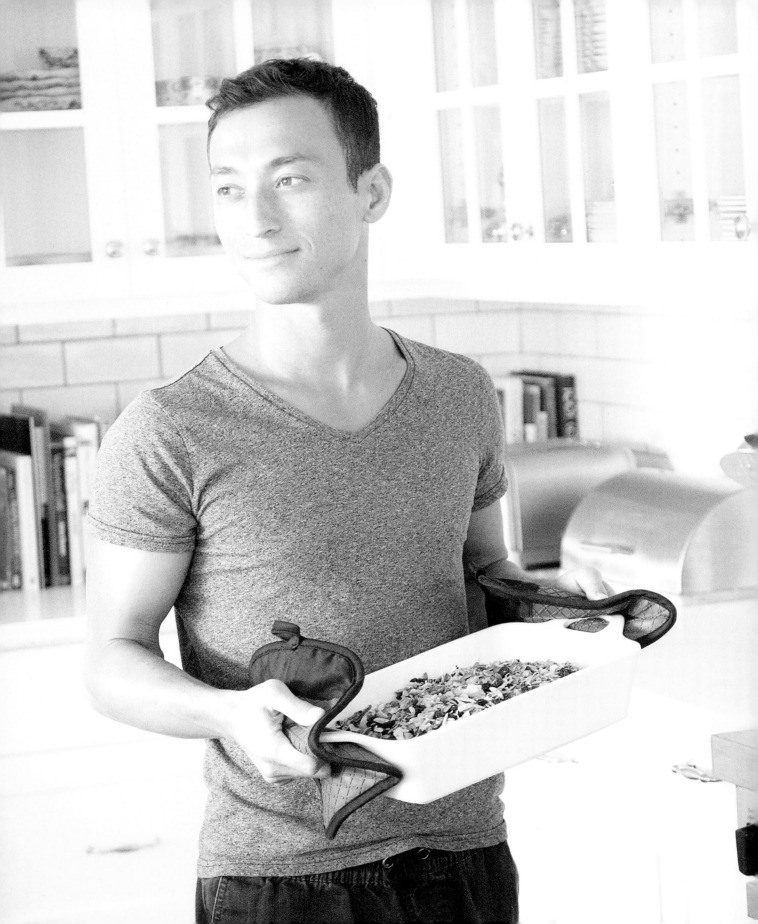

breakfast

Farmhouse Granola

MAKES ABOUT 8 CUPS

Bring that fresh and healthy farmhouse feeling to your breakfast table with this simple, old-fashioned granola recipe. It's full of amazing vitamins, minerals, fiber, and omega-3s, so you'll be ready to head right out to your day after eating a bowlful. It's a perfect after-school snack for your kids, too, or an easy grab-and-go choice for when you're on the run. We tend to have jars of this on hand at all times. At the holidays, we use cranberries in place of the raisins and give it out as presents. After all, homemade gifts are the best—especially ones you can eat! Baking it is a treat, too. It'll make your kitchen smell heavenly. This granola is great all on its own, in a bowl with almond milk, or, Tamal's favorite, on top of coconut ice cream.

2 cups rolled oats

1 cup slivered raw almonds

1 cup raw pecans, coarsely chopped

1 cup raw walnuts, coarsely chopped

1 cup raw pumpkin seeds

½ cup sunflower seeds

¼ cup black sesame seeds

1 cup shredded raw coconut

¼ tsp. Himalayan pink salt

¼ cup melted coconut oil, plus extra for oiling pan

¼ cup maple syrup

¼ cup coconut sugar

1 cup raisins

1 Preheat the oven to 350 degrees F. Using coconut oil, oil a 9x12 glass baking pan.

2 In a large bowl, mix the oats, nuts, seeds, shredded coconut, and salt together until well combined.

3 Stir ¼ cup melted coconut oil into the dry mixture and mix thoroughly. Add the maple syrup and dry coconut sugar and stir well.

4 Spread the mixture in the glass pan and bake for 18 minutes. Remove from oven, stir in the raisins with a spatula, and bake for another 10–12 minutes, until golden brown. Don't bake it for too long, or the raisins will burn.

5 Take out of the oven and let cool for about 30 minutes.

6 Store the granola in a glass jar or airtight container. You can also freeze the granola for up to 4–6 weeks.

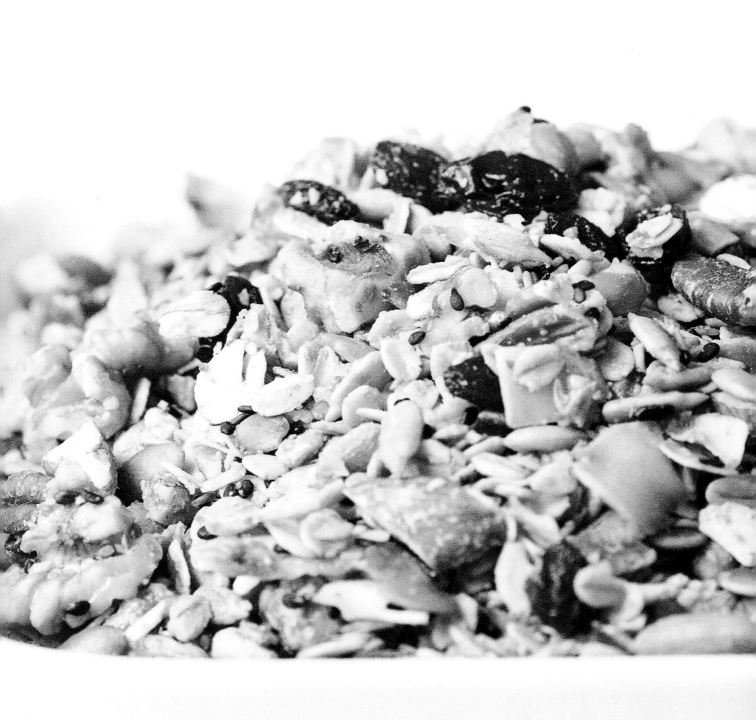

Gramma's Buckwheat Pancakes

Pancakes are so comforting, it's no surprise that millions of people around the world enjoy them day after day. Perhaps you have a memory of your grandmother whipping up some epic goodness in the kitchen and how that warm, moist, fluffy pancake would hit your mouth, syrup dripping from every bite. Or maybe you'd like to make some new memories with the ones you love. Pancakes are a perfect dish to bring people together. We don't usually think of them, however, as a healthy breakfast treat. This recipe is not only delicious but it is packed with whole grains, protein, omega-3s, potassium, and fiber. We like to cover these beautiful, rustic pancakes with coconut yogurt, fresh berries, and some maple syrup.

For the flax egg

1 Tbsp. ground flax meal

3 Tbsp. water

For the pancakes

1 cup buckwheat flour

½ cup white whole-wheat pastry flour

1 tsp. baking soda

1 tsp. cinnamon

2 cups unsweetened nondairy milk (almond, soy, or any nondairy milk you prefer)

1 banana

1 tsp. vanilla extract

Pinch of Himalayan pink salt

Toppings of choice (optional)

1 Mix the flax meal and water in a bowl and set aside until the mixture thickens, about 10 minutes.

1 Place the prepared flax egg and the pancake ingredients in a high-powered blender and blitz until mixed. Ten seconds should be plenty of time — we don't want to overblend.

2 Heat a nonstick skillet and pour the batter into circles of your desired size. We like to make them silver-dollar size and stack them high when they're done. We find they cook really well and are manageable when you don't make them too big. When the pancakes start to bubble on top, it's time to flip them over. As they finish cooking, slide the spatula underneath them and set them onto plates.

3 Top with coconut yogurt and your favorite fruit.

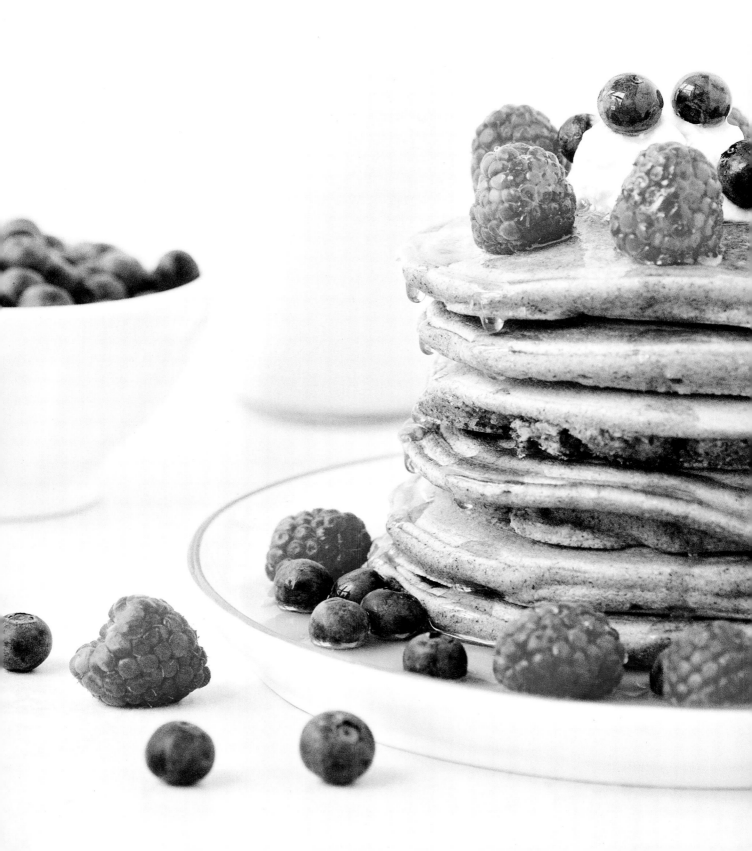

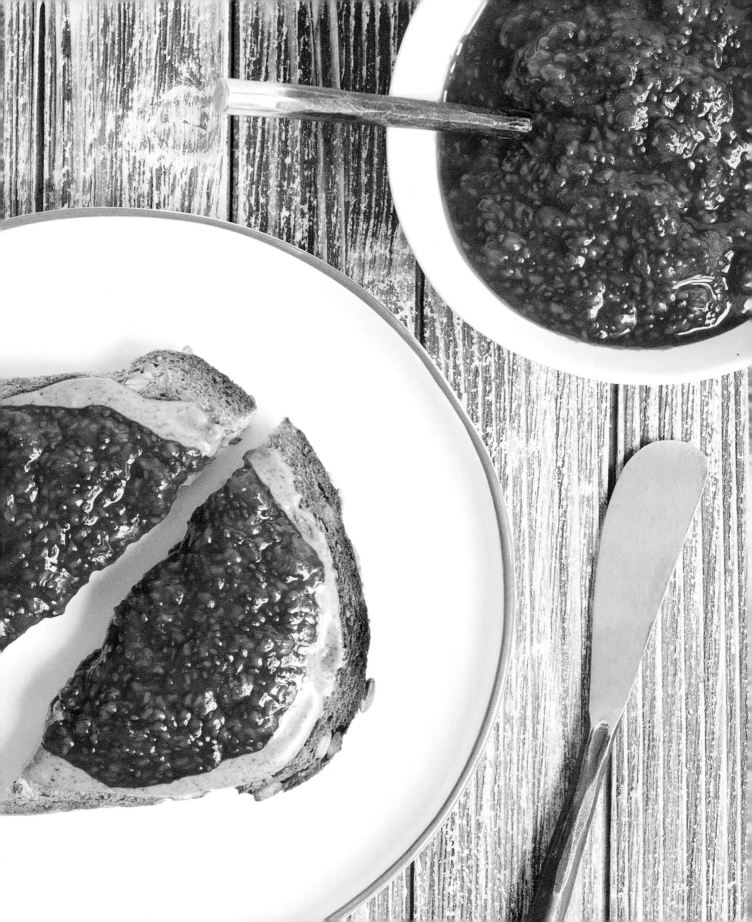

Raspberry Chia Jam

MAKES ABOUT 3 CUPS

There is nothing like homemade jam. It brings that farm-fresh feeling and wholesome goodness right into your kitchen. We enjoy this jam on toast with almond butter (my personal favorite), on top of our Superfood Oatmeal (page 64), in our Cha-Cha-Cha Chia Pudding (page 72), or just about anywhere we want to throw a dollop. This jam is so flavorful, you'll be surprised at how simple it is to make. It's jam-packed (pun intended!) with healthy omegas, fiber, calcium, iron, and antioxidants. For a little variety, it's fun to swap out the raspberries for strawberries, blueberries, or blackberries.

3 cups fresh raspberries (or thawed frozen)

3 Tbsp. maple syrup

3 Tbsp. chia seeds

½ tsp. vanilla extract (optional)

1 In a small pot, bring the raspberries and maple syrup to a low boil, stirring frequently. Reduce the burner to low. Simmer for about 5 minutes, stirring every few minutes.

2 Lightly mash the raspberries with a potato masher or fork, leaving some chunks for texture.

3 Stir in the chia seeds until thoroughly combined. Cook the mixture down for about 15 minutes, until it thickens to your desired consistency. Stir frequently so it doesn't stick to the pot.

4 Once the jam has thickened, remove it from the heat and stir in the vanilla extract.

5 Store in an airtight container in the refrigerator for up to 1 week.

Breakfast Tofu Scramble

SERVES 4

When you need to mix up your breakfast (or even dinner), this dish is the way to go. And it's not just about flavor. This super-high-protein meal will keep your energy soaring for hours. Plus it's packed with iron, vitamin C, calcium, and vitamin B12. We like to serve this with whole-grain toast and fresh tomatoes. Avocado is also a great side. To make the meal extra hearty, whip up some roasted baby potatoes to go with it.

1 19-oz. package firm tofu

1 Tbsp. coconut oil

¼ cup finely chopped red onion

¼ tsp. turmeric powder

¼ tsp. Himalayan pink salt

¼ cup finely chopped red bell pepper

½ cup finely chopped spinach

1 Tbsp. nutritional yeast

Pepper to taste

Fresh cilantro or basil (garnish)

1 Drain the water out of the block of tofu by pressing it in between some paper towels. Squeeze as much of the liquid out as possible. Then crumble the tofu with your hands until it is broken up into tiny pieces.

2 Pour coconut oil into a medium to large sauté pan (cast iron if possible) and turn the burner on to medium heat. Add onion and sauté for about 2–3 minutes, until slightly tender.

3 Add the crumbled tofu and sauté until the water evaporates completely and the tofu is slightly brown. This may take up to 10–15 minutes. Add the turmeric and salt and mix until the tofu is evenly coated. Add bell pepper and spinach and cook until the vegetables are slightly wilted and tender.

4 Add the nutritional yeast right before serving. Season with pepper to taste and garnish with fresh cilantro or basil.

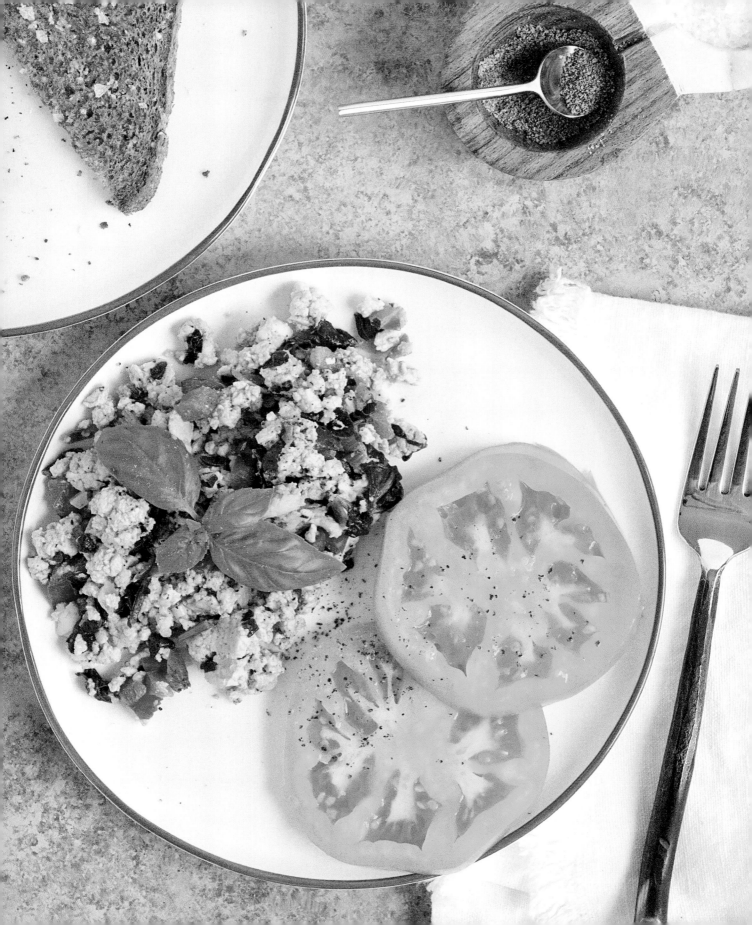

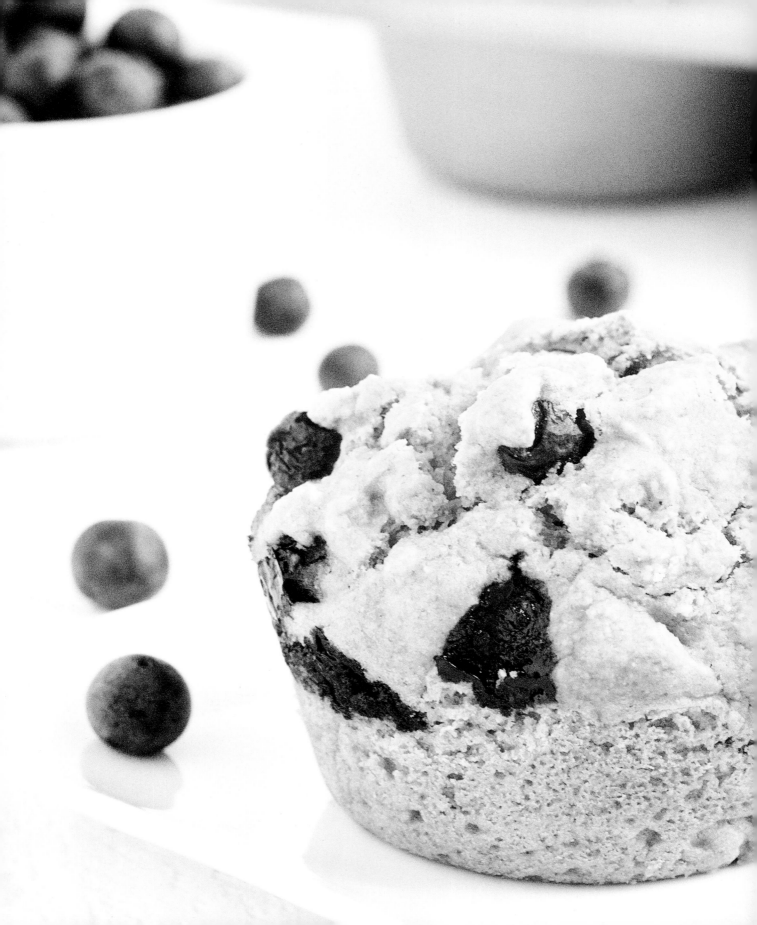

Blissful Blueberry Muffins

MAKES 6 JUMBO OR 12 STANDARD-SIZE MUFFINS

The taste of these muffins might make you feel self-indulgent, but they are full of wholesome ingredients. They're the kind of treat that'll get you through that stretch between meals without any guilt at all. Kids love them, too. They are a crowd pleaser for people of all ages. Drizzle some almond butter or homemade Raspberry Chia Jam (page 59) on them or simply eat them straight up!

2 cups white whole-wheat pastry flour

2 tsp. baking powder

½ tsp. baking soda

½ tsp. Himalayan pink salt

⅓ cup melted coconut oil

1 cup unsweetened nondairy milk

¼ cup unsweetened applesauce

½ cup maple syrup

1 tsp. vanilla extract

1 cup fresh or frozen blueberries

1   Preheat the oven to 350 degrees F. Line a muffin pan with paper liners or lightly grease with coconut oil. (The latter is our favorite method. The muffins pop out of the tin perfectly.)

2   In a medium-size bowl, mix the flour, baking powder, baking soda, and salt together. Add the melted coconut oil to the batter and whisk until blended.

3   In a separate bowl, mix together the nondairy milk, applesauce, maple syrup, and vanilla extract.

4   Combine the dry ingredients and the wet ingredients in one bowl until well blended. Gently fold in the blueberries.

5   Scoop the batter into the muffin cups, filling them about one-third of the way. Bake for 25 minutes. Remove from the oven and let the muffins cool for about 15 minutes.

6   Store in an airtight container for up to 5 days.

Superfood Oatmeal

SERVES 4

Heart-healthy oatmeal has been around for centuries, and for good reason! Yet there's always room for a new spin on a beloved classic. We handpicked a select group of ingredients to give this oatmeal an extra punch of flavor and a hit of superfood quality. Our family eats this oatmeal a few times a week. It's quick, easy, and filling—the perfect meal to start a day.

2 cups rolled oats

1 tsp. cinnamon

⅛ tsp. Himalayan pink salt

1 Tbsp. chia seeds

3 cups water

1 cup unsweetened nondairy milk

1 Tbsp. coconut oil

4 Tbsp. maple syrup

Toppings of choice (optional)

1 Mix the oats, cinnamon, salt, and chia seeds together in a small- to medium-size pot. It is important to combine these ingredients first so that no lumps of cinnamon remain in the oatmeal. Everything should be smoothly and evenly distributed.

2 Add the water and milk to the pot. Cook on medium heat for about 8–10 minutes, stirring occasionally so the oatmeal doesn't stick. Most recipes instruct you to boil water first and then add the oats, but this turns the oats very dry and mushy. The trick to making smooth and creamy oatmeal is to have the oats in the water before you even turn the heat on.

3 Once the oats are done, add the coconut oil and maple syrup and mix well. Pour the oatmeal into bowls and top with blueberries, bananas, coconut flakes, nuts, raisins, or whatever else you like.

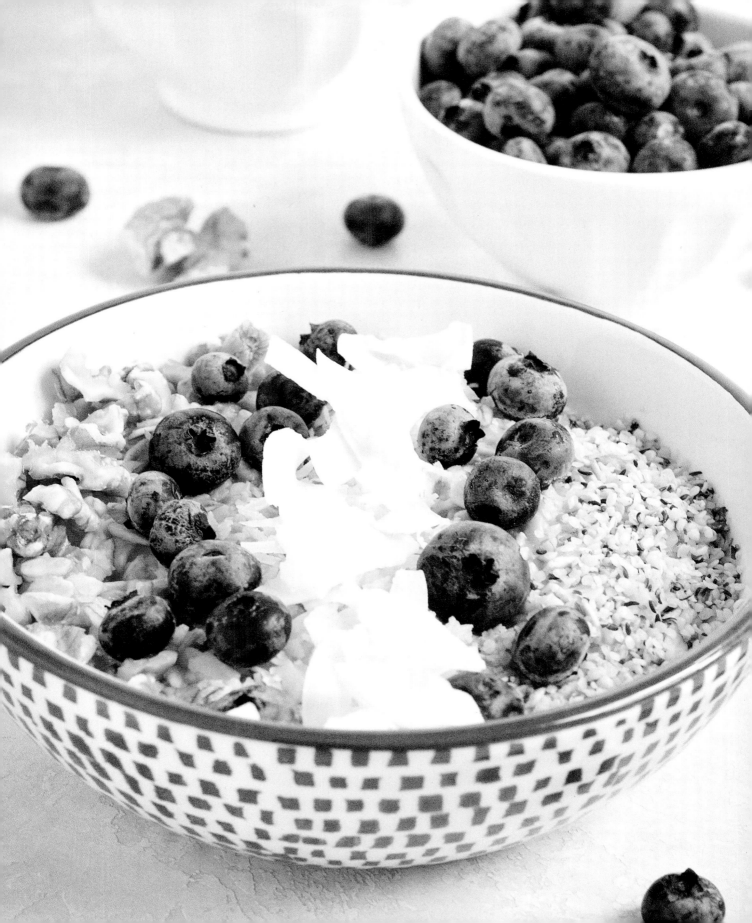

Chickpea Breakfast Crepe

SERVES 4

Our daughter, Savannah, loves a savory breakfast. We often find her exploring the kitchen in the morning, looking for ingredients with which to create a new savory dish for the whole family to enjoy. This recipe celebrates her adventurous spirit in the kitchen. She loves how this Chickpea Breakfast Crepe steps outside the mold of standard vegan scrambled tofu dishes and things of that sort. The crepes are loaded with protein and flavor and will get you ready for the day.

For the batter

1 cup garbanzo bean flour

1 cup water

2 Tbsp. olive oil

½ tsp. baking powder

½ tsp. garlic powder

½ tsp. onion powder

2 Tbsp. nutritional yeast

1 tsp. Himalayan pink salt

⅛ tsp. tumeric

½ cup minced cilantro

For the filling

½ cup diced fresh tomatoes

1 avocado, peeled and sliced

Chopped cilantro

Toppings of choice (optional)

1 Place all the batter ingredients except the cilantro in a high-powered blender and mix for 45 seconds or until well combined.

2 Add in the minced cilantro and blend for another 5–10 seconds, just long enough so that there are only bits of cilantro left.

3 Heat a medium-size nonstick skillet and pour in ⅓ cup of the mixture. Move the pan around so the mixture can spread evenly. Cook over medium heat for 1–2 minutes, or until bubbles form, then flip with a spatula and cook the other side. The crepe should be a light golden brown. Place the crepe on a plate. Repeat until all the crepe batter is used.

4 Fill crepes with tomatoes, avocados, and cilantro. Fold in half and drizzle on top with Magic Tahini Sauce (page 189), Cashew Cream Everything Sauce (page 198), or organic ketchup.

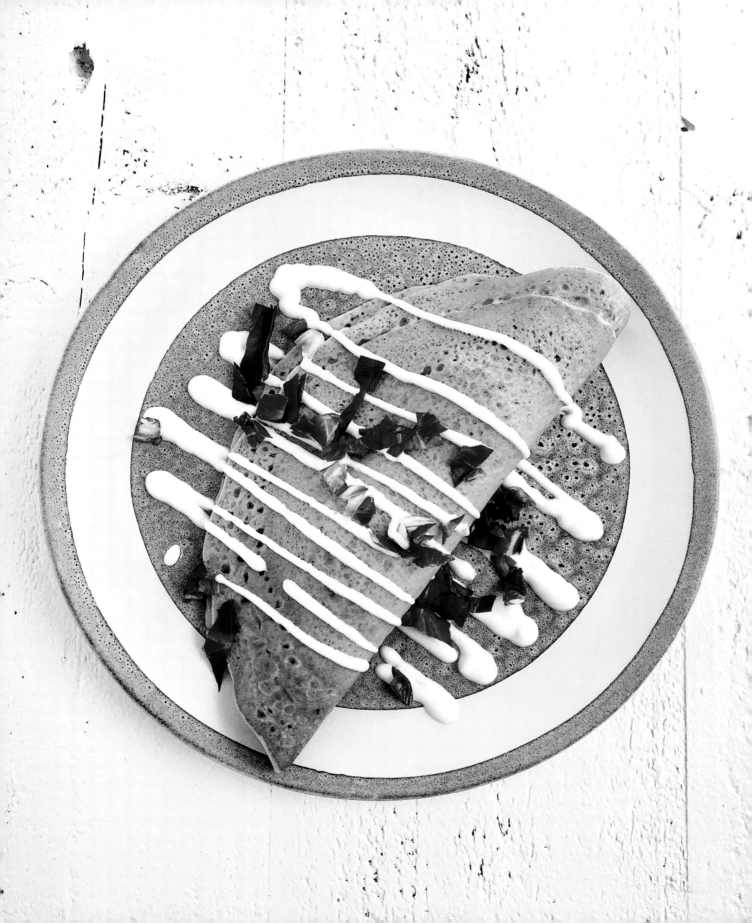

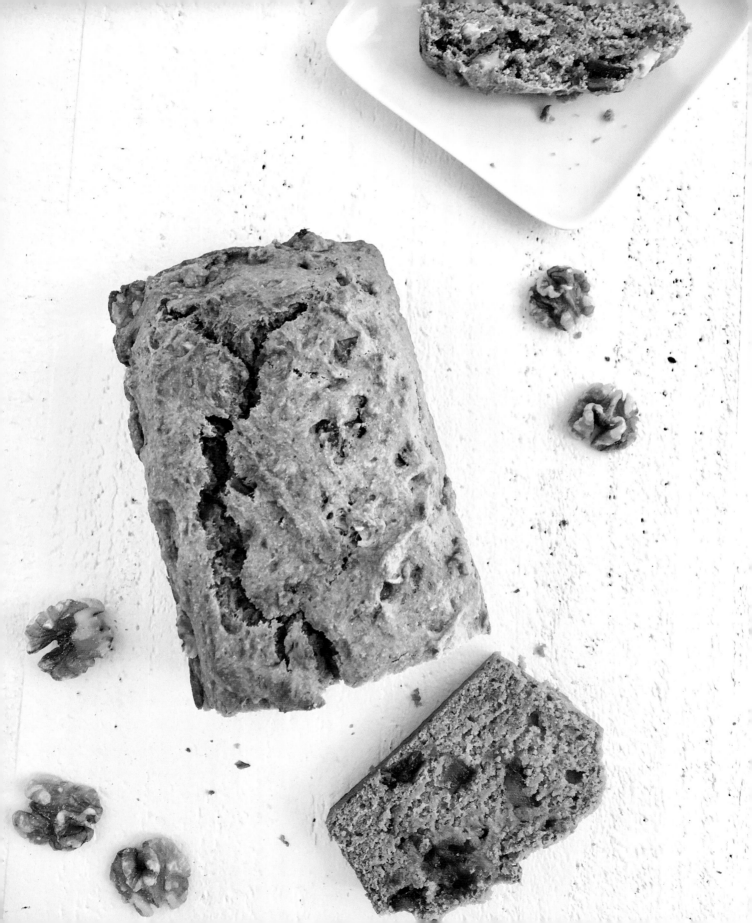

Vegan Banana Walnut Date Bread

MAKES ONE 9-INCH LOAF

This vegan banana bread is bursting with distinctive, mouthwatering flavors. It tastes like dessert, but it will carry you right through the day with its wholesome goodness. It contains fiber, potassium, vitamin E, magnesium, and more. Enjoy a slice right before a long cardio workout. It will give you a steady source of energy and help you push to new limits. Or bring it to a friend's house, and they'll love you forever.

Dry ingredients

1 cup oat flour

1 cup white whole-wheat pastry flour or spelt flour

1 tsp. baking powder

½ tsp. Himalayan pink salt

½ tsp. cinnamon

Wet ingredients

2 mashed ripe bananas

¾ cup coconut sugar

⅓ cup unsweetened almond milk

¼ cup melted coconut oil

2 tsp. vanilla extract

1 flax egg (page 56)

8 chopped dates (preferably Medjool)

¼ cup vegan chocolate chips (optional)

1   Preheat the oven to 375 degrees F. Lightly oil a 9x5 loaf pan with coconut oil.

2   In a medium-size bowl, combine the oat flour, white whole-wheat pastry flour, baking powder, salt, and cinnamon.

3   In a separate bowl, mix together the mashed bananas, coconut sugar, almond milk, melted coconut oil, and vanilla extract, stirring until well combined. Then mix in the flax egg.

4   In a single bowl, combine the wet ingredients with the dry ingredients and stir, being careful not to overstir. Lastly, add the chopped dates and the chocolate chips, if using.

5   Spoon the batter into the loaf pan. Bake the bread for about 35–40 minutes. It's done when a toothpick stuck into the center comes out dry. The top of the bread should be golden brown and slightly firm to the touch.

6   Once out of the oven, lay the loaf pan on its side and let the bread cool for about 30 minutes before serving.

Banana Chocolate Chip Muffins

MAKES 6 JUMBO OR 12 STANDARD-SIZE MUFFINS

Oh, you are in for a treat with these Banana Chocolate Chip Muffins. You'll want them morning, noon, and night. Bursting with fiber, healthy fats, and nourishing vitamins and minerals, these muffins can be served any time of the day. We have them for breakfast with a side of Raw Vanilla Almond Milk (page 39) or as an energy-boosting midday snack. They also make a great after-school treat for the kids.

2¼ cups white whole-wheat pastry flour

2 tsp. baking powder

½ tsp. baking soda

½ tsp. Himalayan pink salt

⅓ cup melted coconut oil

2 mashed ripe bananas

1 cup unsweetened nondairy milk

¼ cup unsweetened applesauce

⅓ cup maple syrup

1 tsp. vanilla extract

½ cup vegan chocolate chips

1. Preheat the oven to 350 degrees F. Line the muffin pan with paper liners or lightly grease the inside of the muffin cups with coconut oil. (The latter is our favorite method. The muffins pop out of the tin perfectly.)

2. In a medium-size bowl, mix together the flour, baking powder, baking soda, and salt. Add the melted coconut oil to the batter and whisk until blended.

3. In a separate bowl, mix together the mashed bananas, nondairy milk, applesauce, maple syrup, and vanilla extract.

4. Mix the dry ingredients together with the wet ingredients. Gently fold in the chocolate chips.

5. Scoop the batter into the muffin cups, filling them about one-third of the way.

6. Bake for 27 minutes. Remove from the oven and let the muffins cool for about 15 minutes.

7. Store in an airtight container for up to 5 days.

Boss French Toast

SERVES 3–4

Breakfast wouldn't be complete without a delicious slice of French toast, fresh out of the pan. Our children love this dish, as it has all the comfort-food components a satisfying breakfast dessert should have. It is sweet, rich, crispy, wholesome, and packed with flavor. Boss French Toast is loaded with healthy fats, protein, and essential nutrients. A few servings of this, and not only will your body function optimally, you'll also have satisfied your guilty cravings! The batter uses nutrient-dense, nonglutinous flour, so you can make this French toast entirely free of gluten if you use gluten-free bread.

1 cup coconut cream

¼ cup unsweetened nondairy milk

2 Tbsp. garbanzo bean flour

2 Tbsp. oat flour

½ tsp. cinnamon

1 Tbsp. maple syrup

1 Tbsp. flax meal

½ tsp. vanilla extract

⅛ tsp. Himalayan pink salt

4–6 slices of bread

½ tsp. coconut oil

Toppings of choice (optional)

1 Heat a nonstick skillet and keep it on medium-low heat while you make the French toast batter. Keeping it warm while you work will save time and energy. The skillet should be hot when you put the toast in it.

2 Place the coconut cream, nondairy milk, two flours, cinammon, maple syrup, flax meal, vanilla extract, and salt in a high-powered blender. Mix until well combined into a batter.

3 Pour the batter into a small baking tray. Dip the slices of bread into the batter, lightly covering both sides and shaking off any excess.

4 Turn the skillet heat up to medium high, add coconut oil to the pan, and carefully lay a slice of the battered French toast in the skillet. Cook for 1–2 minutes on each side, or until it is golden brown. Repeat with the other slices of battered bread.

5 Serve with coconut whipped cream, maple syrup, berries, our Homemade Powdered Sugar (page 214), or anything that inspires you!

Cha-Cha-Cha Chia Pudding

SERVES 2

We tend to make this refreshing, light, and clean dish at night, so that we can wake up the next day, grab it, and go. We're often tempted to eat it as soon as it's ready, though, as it makes a delicious and simple dessert. It's packed with protein and fiber. This is a basic recipe, but there are so many ways to create variations you can always make it seem fresh and new. Start with this version, then you'll want to try some of our favorite combinations, which we've listed below. We like to use our homemade Raw Vanilla Almond Milk (page 39) for the base, but if you don't have that available, you can use unsweetened almond milk. Coconut milk works as a nice, creamy base, too.

1¼ cups unsweetened almond milk

3 Tbsp. chia seeds

¼ tsp. cinnamon

⅛ tsp. vanilla bean powder

1 Tbsp. maple syrup

Toppings of choice (optional)

1 Place all the ingredients in a lidded jar (we like to use a glass mason jar), put the lid on, and shake well until blended. Alternately, you can stir the ingredients together in a bowl, but make sure you stir the chia seeds in well so they don't clump together.

2 Let the mixture stand for 10 minutes and then shake or stir again.

3 Refrigerate for 1 hour or overnight. Store in an airtight container for up to 2–3 days.

4 Serve in bowls and top with berries, granola, chopped almonds, and shredded coconut. Sometimes we like to add cashew or almond butter to make it even heartier. So good!

For variations, you can add 1 Tbsp. cacao powder, ¼ cup frozen blueberries, ½ tsp. lemon or orange zest, or ⅛ tsp. cardamom plus ½ tsp. cinnamon.

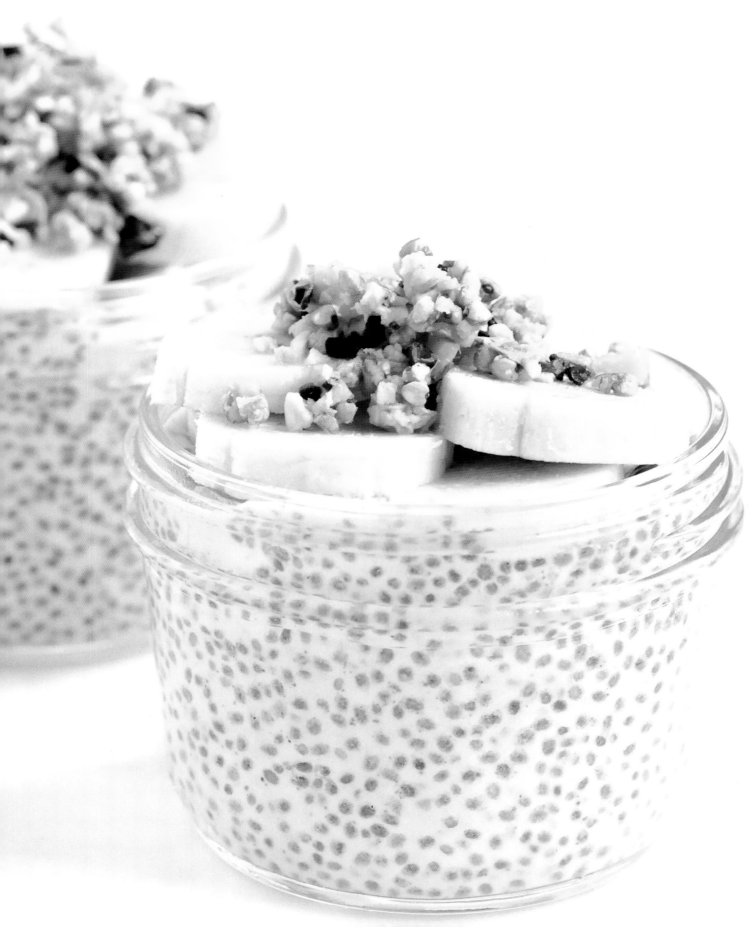

Chocolate Raspberry Muffins

MAKES 6 JUMBO OR 12 STANDARD-SIZE MUFFINS

When we were thinking about which muffins to include in this book, we knew we couldn't do without this recipe. It's a fan favorite among family and friends. The flavors complement one another perfectly: the creamy chocolate and fresh sweetness, along with a little bit of tartness, from the raspberry. The texture of these muffins—crispy tops and moist centers—will take your senses to another level. We love to whip up a batch early in the morning and start the day off with a warm, cozy vibe. Top them off with our Whipped Cream from Heaven (page 204), and you'll be transported to heaven with every bite.

2 cups white whole-wheat pastry flour

2 tsp. baking powder

½ tsp. baking soda

½ tsp. Himalayan pink salt

1 cup unsweetened almond milk

¼ cup unsweetened applesauce

½ cup maple syrup

1 tsp. vanilla extract

⅓ cup coconut oil

1 cup fresh or frozen raspberries

½ cup mini vegan chocolate chips

1 Preheat the oven to 350 degrees F. Line the muffin pan with paper liners or lightly grease the inside of the muffin cups with coconut oil. (The latter is our favorite method. The muffins pop out of the tin perfectly.)

2 In a medium-size bowl, sift together the flour, baking powder, baking soda, and salt. The sifting ensures there will be no clumps in the batter.

3 In a separate bowl, mix together the almond milk, applesauce, maple syrup, and vanilla extract.

4 In a small pot, heat the coconut oil until it is melted. Do not skip this part. If you add room-temperature coconut oil, the wet mixture will not be smooth, and the muffins will be clumpy. Once melted, add coconut oil to the other wet ingredients and mix well.

5 Mix the dry ingredients together with the wet ingredients. Gently fold in the raspberries and chocolate chips. If you are using frozen raspberries, make sure they are at room temperature when tossing in.

6 Scoop the batter into the muffin cups, filling them about one-third of the way. Bake for 25–27 minutes. Remove from the oven and let the muffins cool for about 10–15 minutes.

7 Store in an airtight container for up to 5 days.

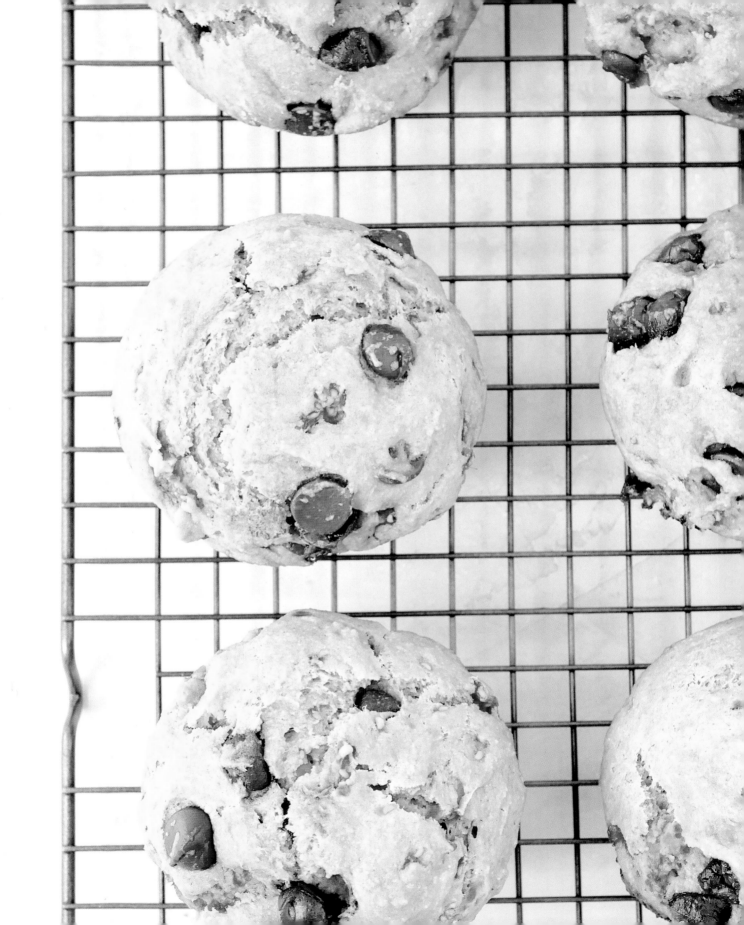

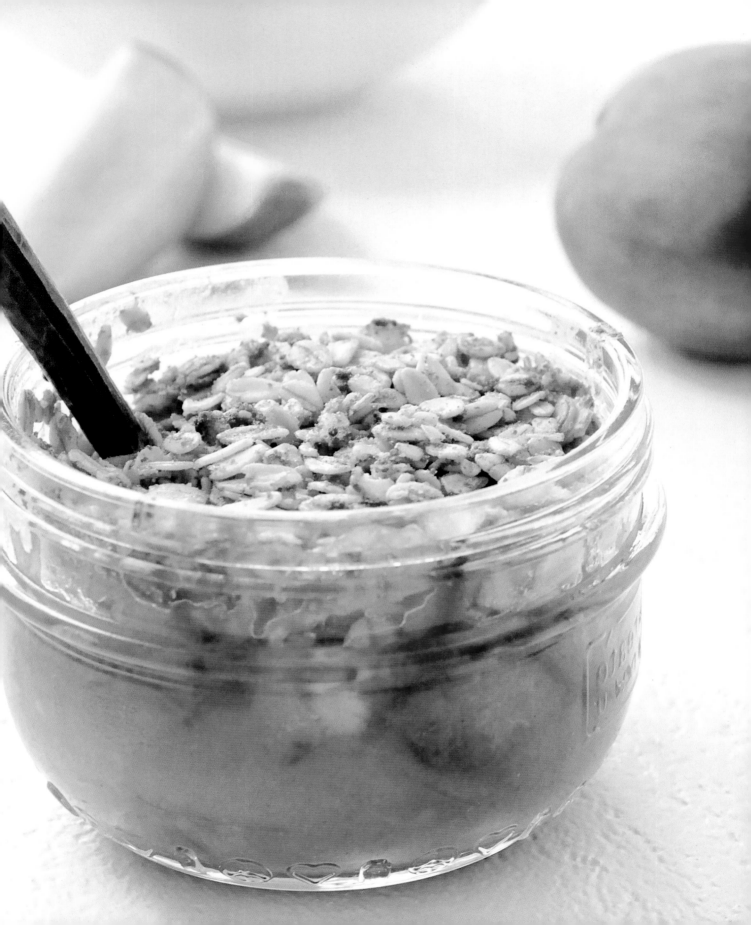

Mason Jar Peach Crisp Crumble

MAKES FOUR 8-OZ. JARS

We all love the idea of dessert for breakfast, but rarely is that a healthy choice, as we don't want to start our day with refined sugars and refined grains. But when you eat this Peach Crisp first thing in the morning, it'll only *taste* like you are breaking the rules. Our farm-style breakfast dish is healthy, filling, and good for you. It is loaded with good fats, unrefined sugar, and whole grains. We bake it in individual glass jars to make it easy to serve. This is the kind of meal that'll make you happy to hear the alarm first thing in the morning!

For the filling

4 cups pitted and chopped fresh peaches (or thawed frozen)

1 Tbsp. arrowroot powder

¼ cup maple syrup

1 Tbsp. lemon juice

Pinch of Himalayan pink salt

½ tsp. vanilla extract

½ tsp. cinnamon

¼ tsp. ginger powder

For the topping

½ cup rolled oats

½ cup spelt flour

¼ tsp. cinnamon

4 Tbsp. melted coconut oil

¼ tsp. Himalayan pink salt

3 Tbsp. coconut sugar

¼ cup pecans

1   Preheat the oven to 375 degrees F.

2   Place the chopped peaches, arrowroot powder, maple syrup, lemon juice, salt, vanilla extract, cinnamon, and ginger powder in a large bowl and mix until combined.

3   In a separate bowl, mix the topping ingredients together well.

4   Fill one 8-oz. glass jar three-quarters of the way with peach filling. Add one-fourth of the topping mixture on top. Repeat this process with three other 8-oz. glass jars.

5   Bake in the oven for 15–20 minutes. Let cool for about 5–8 minutes and enjoy!

Mexican Breakfast Hash

SERVES 4

Breakfast is the most important meal of the day and should fill you with hearty, nutrient-dense fuel that will keep you going strong. This Mexican Breakfast Hash was created by Tamal to honor his fond memories of the delicious Mexican food his mother would make when he was a child. His family used to devour large plates of black beans, tortillas, salsa, and Mexican potato enchiladas. Tamal set out to design a dish that will make you feel good during the day, but also has the comforting qualities of dinner — and so this Mexican Breakfast Hash was born! It is tangy, spicy, salty, and filling.

For the sauce

1 guajillo chile pepper, stemmed and deseeded

1 chile de arbol, stemmed and deseeded

1 pasilla chile pepper, stemmed and deseeded

2 bay leaves

½ tsp. cumin

½ tsp. oregano

½ tsp. paprika

1 Tbsp. apple cider vinegar

1 Tbsp. white sesame seeds

1 Tbsp. maple syrup

3 allspice berries

½ cup diced tomato

1 Tbsp. olive oil

½ cup chopped cilantro

¼ cup vegan mayonnaise, such as Vegenaise

½ tsp. Himalayan pink salt

1 Cook the guajillo, arbol, and pasilla peppers in a pot of boiling water for 2–3 minutes, or until tender.

2 Drain the peppers and put them in a food processor with the rest of the sauce ingredients. Process until mixed well (about 75 percent blended), stopping occasionally to scrape down the sides of the food processor with a spatula. Leaving the mixture slightly chunky gives it character and prevents it from becoming a dressing.

For the filling

2 Tbsp. coconut
oil, for cooking

1 cup diced russet potato
(¼-inch pieces)

½ cup diced onion

1 cup minced mushrooms

½ cup diced walnuts

¼ tsp. Himalayan pink salt

To serve

Tortillas

Toppings of choice (optional)

1 Heat 1 Tbsp. of the coconut oil in a skillet and add
the diced potatoes, sautéing until they are golden
brown and tender. Transfer the potatoes to a bowl
and set aside.

2 Add another 1 Tbsp. of coconut oil to the skillet plus
the onions, cooking them until they are tender.
Throw in the mushrooms and sauté until they are
nice and soft.

3 Add the chopped walnuts to the onions and
mushrooms. Sauté the mixture for 2–3
more minutes.

4 Then add the chile sauce, cooked potatoes,
and ¼ tsp. salt. Mix well.

5 Serve on a plate with tortillas, Cashew Cream
Everything Sauce (page 198), sliced avocados,
and salsa. Everyone can make their own
stuffed tortillas.

Classic Zucchini Bread

MAKES ONE 9-INCH LOAF

When we're craving breakfast bread, we're yearning for one of those lightly sweet, wholesome staples, like banana bread, cranberry orange bread, pumpkin bread, or our household favorite, zucchini bread. A filling energy booster, our Classic Zucchini Bread is infused with vegetables, whole grains, and good fats. This is a slightly sweet, moist, and hearty variation that has all the classic flavors but adds a plethora of health components into the mix. It is both nourishing and comforting, a perfect way to start the day.

Dry ingredients

2 cups white whole-wheat pastry flour

¾ cup coconut sugar

1 tsp. baking soda

1 tsp. baking powder

1 tsp. cinnamon

1 tsp. Himalayan pink salt

Wet ingredients

1 cup shredded zucchini

½ cup unsweetened applesauce

1 cup unsweetened nondairy milk

¼ cup almond butter

¼ cup melted coconut oil

1 Tbsp. apple cider vinegar

1 flax egg (page 56)

½ tsp. vanilla extract

¼ cup chopped walnuts (garnish)

1 Preheat the oven to 350 degrees F. Oil a 9x5 loaf pan and set it aside.

2 Sift all the dry ingredients together in a large bowl to eliminate lumps and mix well.

3 In a separate bowl, combine all the wet ingredients and stir well.

4 Combine the wet and dry ingredients in one bowl and fold together until they are well mixed.

5 Pour the batter into the oiled loaf pan and garnish with chopped walnuts. Bake in the oven for 45 minutes, or until a toothpick in the center comes out clean.

6 Serve with your favorite vegan butter.

Creamy Homemade Coconut Yogurt

SERVES 3–4

This yogurt takes a bit of effort to make, but it is worth the time, and you will cherish and savor every bite. Cracking the coconuts and cleaning out the meat takes the majority of the labor, but with a little practice, you can speed up the process. Most recently, when Victoria timed herself, it took only 20 minutes to clean three coconuts. Not too bad. The health benefits from coconuts are immense. They are antibacterial, antiparasitic, and antifungal. Coconuts are loaded with vitamin E. They increase your energy with medium-chain fatty acids, in addition to improving your digestion and speeding up the healing process when you're under the weather. Coconut water also contains electrolytes, so it's particularly beneficial after a workout. And that's just the short list of coconut's strengths. Needless to say, this is a very nourishing dish.

2–3 young Thai coconuts

1 Tbsp. maple syrup

1 capsule or ¼ tsp. probiotic powder

⅛ tsp. vanilla bean powder (optional, but highly recommended)

For easy-to-follow visuals on opening a coconut, see the tutorial video "How to Open a Coconut" on Victoria's The Yoga Plate YouTube channel.

1. To open the coconuts: Place a coconut on its side. Shave the husks off the top point with a very sharp knife. Whack the sharp edge of the knife around the top of the coconut until you form a circle. Pry it open with a butter knife, pour the coconut water into a glass or jar, and scoop the coconut meat out with a spoon. Rinse the meat well.

2. Place 2 cups coconut meat, maple syrup, and ½ cup coconut water into a high-speed blender and process until smooth. It may take several minutes to get the coconut smooth.

3. Pour the mixture into a medium-size bowl and stir in the probiotic and vanilla bean powders.

4. Cover with a clean kitchen towel and leave out on your counter overnight. In the morning you will have your finished product! You can top with fresh mango and strawberries or berries and granola. The possibilities are endless.

5. Store in an airtight container or mason jars for up to 1 week (if it lasts that long!).

Mashed Peas on Toast

SERVES 4

This is a refreshing, light breakfast that's packed with protein and nutrients. You'd be surprised at how flavorful such a simple dish can be! Our family loves to eat this on hot summer afternoons or when we need a little extra color in our lives, as it looks so pretty.

2 Tbsp. olive oil

2 Tbsp. minced red onion

1 tsp. minced garlic

1½ cups frozen green peas

½ tsp. Himalayan pink salt

2 Tbsp. lemon juice

4 slices of bread, toasted

Olive oil (for drizzling)

Zest of 1 lemon (garnish)

Red chili flakes
(optional garnish)

1 Heat the olive oil in a small pot, then add the onions and garlic. Sauté over medium heat for 2–3 minutes, or until the onions are soft, then add the frozen peas and salt. Cook for another 5 minutes, or until the peas are soft. Stir in lemon juice and cook for 2 minutes more.

2 Turn the heat off and mash the peas with a potato masher or transfer to a food processor and blend. If you use a food processor, stop occasionally and scrape the sides down with a spatula to get an even blend. But leave some of the peas chunky — you don't want to create a puree.

3 Spread the mashed peas on the slices of toast and drizzle with olive oil. Sprinkle each with a pinch of lemon zest and red chili flakes, if using.

Sugar-Free, Gluten-Free Lemon Poppy Seed Scones

MAKES ABOUT 8 SCONES

People often think of vegans as hippie, salad-eating, tree-hugging, granola-munching yogis. The funny thing is, we really do love all of those things, but we aren't limited to them. We eat much more than granola and salad in our house. We enjoy baking, and scones are one of our favorite breakfast treats. Complement these with our Raspberry Chia Jam (page 59) and a warm almond milk tea. This classic recipe has been altered so that it is sugar free and gluten free, but certainly not flavor free!

2 cups all-purpose gluten-free baking flour, such as Bob's Red Mill

1 Tbsp. baking powder

3 Tbsp. xylitol

½ tsp. Himalayan pink salt

1 Tbsp. poppy seeds

½ cup melted coconut oil

¼ cup unsweetened nondairy milk

1 Tbsp. lemon juice

Zest of 1 lemon

1 tsp. vanilla extract

1. Preheat the oven to 400 degrees F. Line a medium-size baking sheet with parchment paper.

2. In a large bowl, mix together the flour, baking powder, xylitol, salt, and poppy seeds until well combined.

3. Add coconut oil and mix in well, then add nondairy milk, lemon juice, lemon zest, and vanilla extract. Combine thoroughly.

4. Turn the dough out onto a cutting board dusted with flour. Gently knead the dough and form it into a circle about ½ inch thick. Cut into triangular pieces, like pie slices.

5. Lay the scones on the baking sheet lined with parchment paper. With a baking brush, lightly coat the tops of the scones with a little nondairy milk. Sprinkle each with a pinch of xylitol.

6. Bake for 12–15 minutes, until the bottoms of the scones are light golden brown in color. Let the scones cool for about 5–8 minutes and then serve.

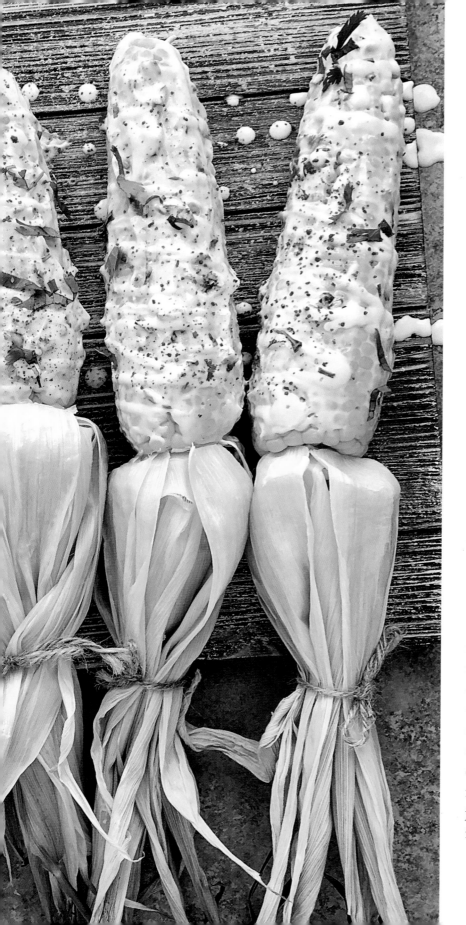

plate full of prana

In the yogic tradition, *prana* means "life energy." This doesn't just refer to the air we breathe but also to the prana we take in through food, water, the sun, and the people we surround ourselves with. When we are feeling low on energy, we need to make sure the food and drinks we consume are optimized to revitalize our system. The recipes in this section can serve as quick, easy, delicious lunches or midday snacks that are jam-packed with energizing ingredients.

snacks and sides

Prana Power Bar

MAKES 24 BITE-SIZE PIECES

We spend a lot of our busy lives on the go, dashing from one place to the next. It can be challenging to find a healthy snack to keep our energy up. These bite-size Prana Power Bars are perfect for when you're on the move. Try one just before your workout or right after—they'll power you up without making you feel too full. These chocolate beauties have many health benefits: fiber, antioxidants, heart-healthy fats, vitamin C, and lots of minerals, just to name a few. We store them in the freezer and then move half a dozen or so to the fridge so that they're ready when we need them. The kids love them too as an after-school snack. Who turns down chocolate, after all?

For the dough

1 cup almonds

1½ cups rolled oats

½ cup coconut oil

½ cup shredded unsweetened coconut

¼ cup cacao powder

¼ cup maple syrup

¼ cup goji berries

¼ cup mulberries

¼ cup chia seeds

¼ tsp. Himalayan pink salt

For the chocolate sauce

½ cup vegan chocolate chips

2 tsp. coconut oil

Pinch of Himalayan pink salt

1 Soak 1 cup of almonds in water overnight or for at least 2–3 hours, until soft.

2 In a food processor combine the soaked almonds, oats, coconut oil, shredded coconut, cacao powder, and maple syrup. Pulse until a dough forms.

3 Add the goji berries, mulberries, chia seeds, and salt and process again until everything is well mixed.

4 Take a spoonful of batter and press into a silicone mold (we use a mold that has 1x1-inch squares, but any small shape works) or mini cupcake liner. Flatten out the top. Repeat until you have used all the batter. Freeze for about 1 hour.

5 In a small pot, heat the chocolate chips, coconut oil, and salt until the mixture becomes liquid.

6 Line a baking sheet or large platter with parchment paper. Remove a bar from its mold or cupcake liner and dip one side into the chocolate sauce, then lay it on the parchment paper. Continue until all the bars are half-covered in chocolate.

7 Place in the freezer again until the chocolate hardens, about 30 minutes.

8 Store in an airtight container in the freezer or refrigerator for up to 1 week.

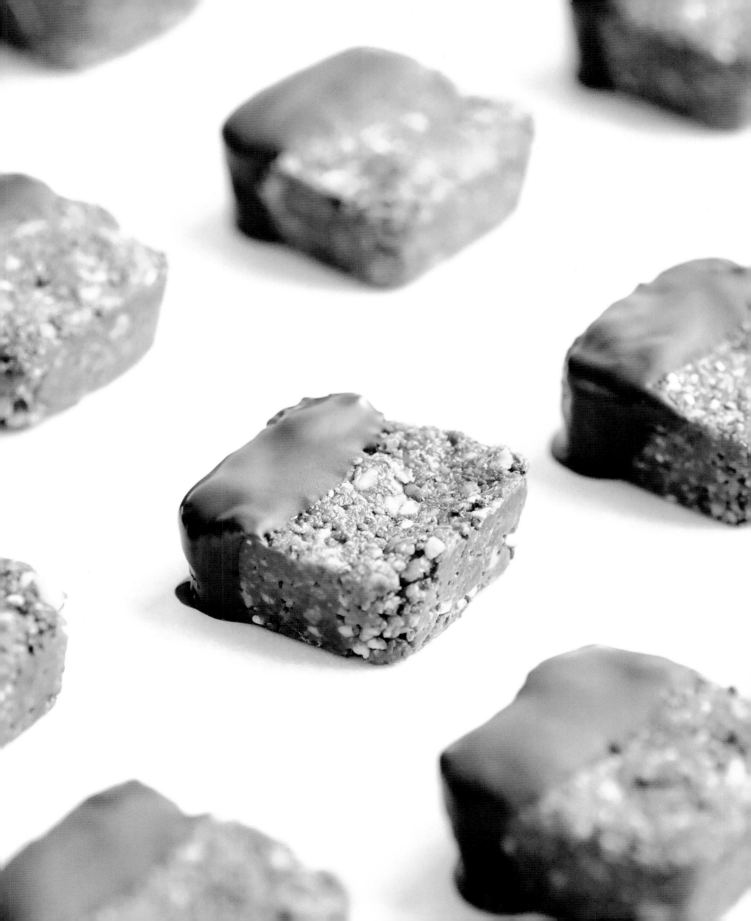

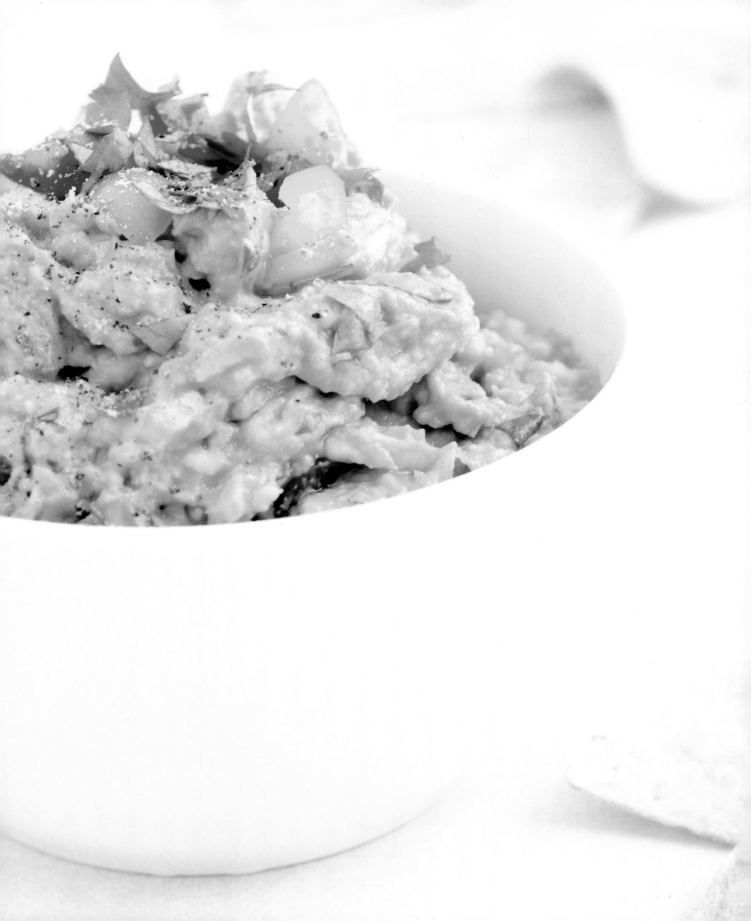

Holy Mole Guacamole!

MAKES ABOUT 2 CUPS

Guacamole is a universally loved food. I associate it with good times and coming together with people we love. We bring this dish to family dinners, picnics, and game day, and of course it is something we enjoy on our own. Our family can eat this whole recipe in one sitting and still crave more! This version carries those classic creamy and salty flavors that we look for in a rich guacamole.

3 medium-size ripe avocados, peeled, pitted, and cut into chunks

¼ cup finely diced tomato

1 Tbsp. diced red onion

½ tsp. minced garlic

½ tsp. Himalayan pink salt

3 Tbsp. lime juice

1 Tbsp. minced cilantro

1   Place avocados in a medium bowl and mash them well. Our family likes to keep little chunks of avocado in so that the guacamole isn't too mushy.

2   Mix in the diced tomato, red onion, garlic, salt, and lime juice.

3   Lastly, fold in the cilantro. Serve with tortilla chips.

Movie Nacho Cheese

MAKES ABOUT 2 CUPS

Do you remember getting nachos at a movie theater or a ballpark when you were growing up? Carrying that tray of steaming hot chips to your seat, with cheese that is creamy, salty, and tangy in all the right ways? Maybe you've avoided indulging in this decadent snack since then. We've crafted a variation that is all pleasure and no guilt. It's packed with vegetables and nutrients, and it'll still evoke those childhood memories, because it tastes so good.

1 cup cubed white potatoes

½ cup cubed carrots

¼ cup grape-seed oil

¼ cup water

2 tsp. lemon juice

4 pickled jalapeño slices

2 Tbsp. jalapeño pickle juice

2 tsp. arrowroot flour

1 tsp. garlic powder

1 tsp. onion powder

1 Tbsp. nutritional yeast

⅛ tsp. turmeric powder

½ tsp. Himalayan pink salt

Corn chips

Toppings of choice (optional)

1 Cook the cubed potatoes and carrots in a pot of boiling water for 10–15 minutes, or until soft.

2 Drain the carrots and potatoes and place them in a high-powered blender as soon as they are out of the water. Add all the remaining ingredients to the blender and process until smooth and creamy.

3 Drizzle warm over corn chips and then top with guacamole, black beans, and salsa.

This cheese is also great poured over homemade veggie pizza as a substitute for store-bought vegan cheese.

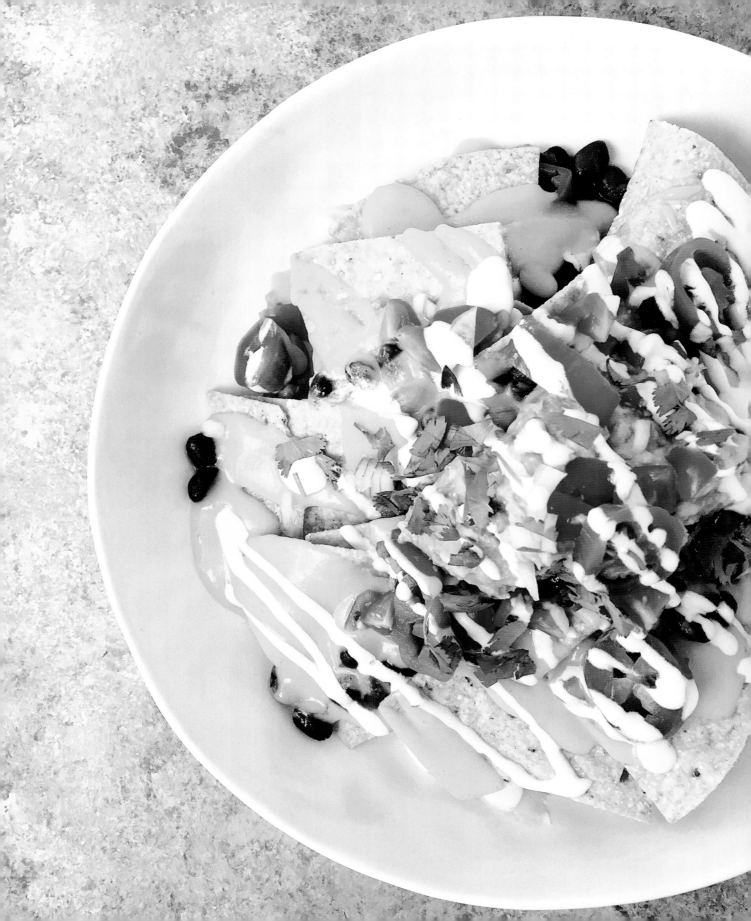

Elote (Mexican Street Corn)

SERVES 3–4

Corn on the cob is always a classic side that complements all sorts of dishes. You can have it with mashed potatoes and gravy in the winter or with veggie burgers and coleslaw at a summer dinner. Corn is enjoyed by cultures around the world, and they all have developed different ways to prepare it. *Elote* is a corn-on-the-cob dish from Mexico. It is creamy, sour, spicy, and decadent, and it's often eaten as a late-night snack. We love this simple recipe in our house and eat it as an appetizer with any Mexican-inspired meal.

4–6 ears of corn

¼ cup vegan mayonnaise, such as Vegenaise

¼ cup Cashew Cream Everything Sauce (page 198)

2 Tbsp. minced cilantro

2 Tbsp. lime juice

¼ tsp. Himalayan pink salt

¼ tsp. chili powder

¼ tsp. onion powder

¼ tsp. garlic powder

Toppings of choice (optional)

1 In a large pot, steam 4–6 ears of corn until tender and set aside.

2 In a small bowl, mix together the vegan mayonnaise, Cashew Cream Everything Sauce, cilantro, lime juice, salt, chili powder, onion powder, and garlic powder.

3 Smother each ear of corn with some of the sauce. Sprinkle with cashews, grated vegan Parmesan, and minced cilantro if you wish, or just serve by itself.

Kanai's Mac & Cheese

SERVES 4

Let's face it: mac & cheese is just about the most nostalgic dish out there for many of us. It brings us back to a time when our priorities were completely different. Playing hard with our friends was at the top of the list. And good, hearty food was part of that joy. This recipe captures that time, and it can define that joy for a whole new generation. Our kids love this mac & cheese, so much so that our son, Kanai, asked that we add it to the weekly menu. We're happy to say yes, because this version is loaded with veggies in the secret sauce. So it's packed with the good stuff and still tastes like the guilty stuff!

1 16-oz. package whole-wheat or gluten-free macaroni noodles

3 cups diced potatoes

½ cup diced carrots

¼ cup cashews, soaked for at least 2 hours

2¼ tsp. Himalayan pink salt

2 Tbsp. lemon juice

½ tsp. garlic powder

½ tsp. onion powder

2 Tbsp. olive oil

4 Tbsp. nutritional yeast

⅛ tsp. turmeric powder

1 Follow the cooking instructions on the package of macaroni noodles and set them aside.

2 Boil potatoes and carrots in a pot of water until soft, about 10–15 minutes. Drain the potatoes and carrots, reserving 1 cup of broth.

3 Place the potatoes, carrots, and reserved broth in a high-powered blender and blend until smooth. We like to do this while the potatoes, carrots, and broth are still really hot, so that they mash more easily and the end result is that melted, creamy mac & cheese texture.

4 Add in the soaked cashews, salt, lemon juice, garlic powder, onion powder, olive oil, nutritional yeast, and turmeric. Blend at high speed for 45 seconds twice, or until the mixture is creamy and smooth.

5 Serve over the macaroni noodles right away, while the sauce is still warm.

Classic Hummus

MAKES ABOUT 2 CUPS

This truly is the most delicious and easy-to-make recipe in the world. Throw everything into the blender and voilà! Use it for a sandwich spread, a dip for raw veggies, or a spread for just plain old pitas. It's a great source of plant-based protein that even kids love.

1½ cups cooked organic garbanzo beans

½ cup tahini

3 Tbsp. olive oil

1 garlic clove, peeled

½ cup fresh lemon juice

¼ cup water

¾ tsp. Himalayan pink salt

Pepper to taste

Suggested toppings

Paprika

Parsley sprigs

Toasted pine nuts

Drizzle of olive oil

1 Put all of the ingredients into a food processor or blender and blend until smooth, stopping to scrape down the sides with a spatula as needed. This may need several rounds of processing to get smooth.

2 Top with paprika, parsley, toasted pine nuts, and a drizzle of olive oil, and you will have a beautiful side.

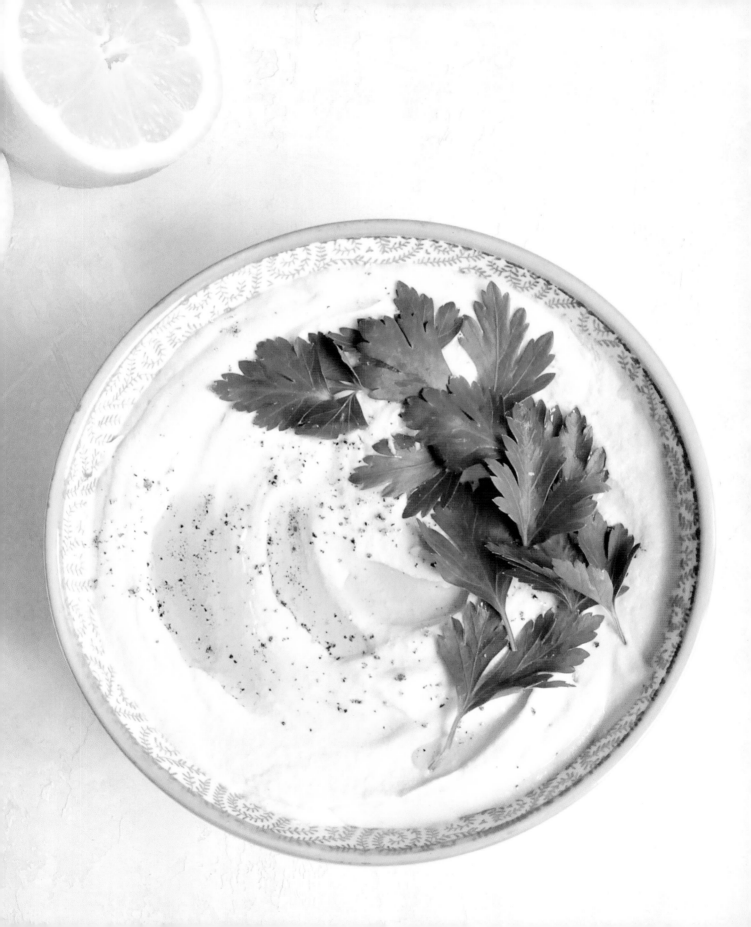

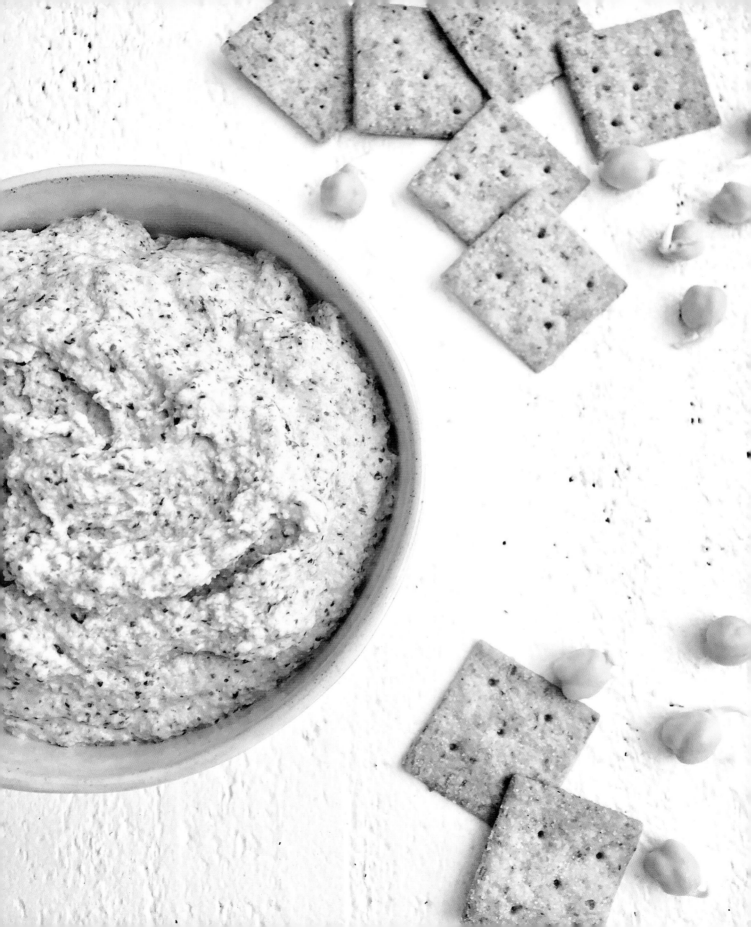

Sprouted Cilantro Jalapeño Hummus

MAKES 3½ CUPS

This hummus is an energetic superfood. When you soak and sprout any seed or legume, its nutrients more than double, and it becomes a "live" food. Consumed in a raw state, the sprouted seeds deliver enzymes and micronutrients that would be destroyed if cooked. This hummus is bursting with protein, fiber, heart-healthy fats, and heavy-metal-cleansing cilantro. You could sustain yourself for hours with high levels of energy from this dip. For all that it delivers, it still tastes light and fresh. It makes a perfect summer picnic dip for crackers or a spread for a pita on a hot day, postworkout. Or simply drop a dollop on the side of a Mediterranean salad.

2 cups dry garbanzo beans

1 garlic clove, peeled

1 jalapeño pepper

½ cup olive oil

6 Tbsp. lemon juice

1 tsp. Himalayan pink salt

1 cup cilantro

4 Tbsp. flax meal

1 tsp. cumin

To sprout the garbanzo beans

1 Place the garbanzo beans in a bowl of water with at least 2 inches of water above the beans. Soak at least 8 hours or overnight.

2 Drain the water and rinse the garbanzo beans thoroughly. Then place in a colander or strainer and cover with a very light towel or paper towel. Every 8 hours, remove the towel, rinse the beans, and cover again. Repeat for about 24 hours, until you see little tails form at the tips of the beans. The longer the beans sprout, the sweeter they will become.

To make the hummus

1 Place the garlic clove in a food processor and mince.

2 Add the sprouted garbanzo beans, jalapeño, olive oil, lemon juice, and salt. Process until smooth.

3 Add in the cilantro, flax meal, and cumin. Process again.

4 Store in an airtight container for up to 1 week.

Cauliflower Mash

SERVES 4–6

Mashed potatoes can be delicious and wholesome, and this dish proves it. Cauliflower Mash is a healthy alternative to standard mashed potatoes, and your kids won't even notice the difference. The creamy potatoes and the crunchy cauliflower are a winning combination. This side dish is low in carbs, high in fiber, and loaded with vitamin C, along with many other vitamins and minerals, such as potassium and magnesium. We love to eat Cauliflower Mash year-round in our house. It's a no-brainer in our book.

3 medium-size baking potatoes

1 small cauliflower head

½ cup vegan mayonnaise, such as Vegenaise

Salt and pepper to taste

Finely chopped chives (garnish)

1   Wash the potatoes well. Peel the potatoes and chop them into large chunks about 1½–2 inches thick.

2   Place the potatoes in a large pot and fill with water. Bring to a boil and cook for about 10–12 minutes.

3   While the potatoes are boiling, destem and chop the cauliflower. Add the cauliflower to the potatoes and boil for another 10–15 minutes, until the vegetables are tender.

4   Drain the vegetables into a strainer, then place them back in the pot. With a potato masher, mash the mixture well.

5   Add the vegan mayonnaise and salt and pepper to taste and blend well. The dish should be smooth and creamy.

6   Transfer to a serving bowl or to individual plates. Top it off with some finely chopped chives and serve with Shiitake Holiday Gravy (page 203).

American *Farinata*

MAKES 1 MEDIUM-SIZE SKILLET BREAD

Farinata is a light, nutritious, gluten-free bread that is enjoyed in Italy. We've modified the traditional style and call our version American *Farinata*. We added corn flour (masa), so that the bread has a hint of corn bread flavor. It's also fluffier than the original, because we've added baking powder. This dish pairs well with the Magic Tahini Sauce (page 189) or the Cashew Cream Everything Sauce (page 198). We also like to pour salad greens over our American *Farinata* and douse with salad dressing.

½ cup masa flour
(we use Bob's Red Mill)

½ cup garbanzo bean flour

½ tsp. baking powder

½ tsp. Himalayan pink salt

½ tsp. oregano

½ tsp. thyme

1 Tbsp. olive oil

1 Tbsp. maple syrup

1 Tbsp. olive oil (for baking)

1   Preheat the oven to 450 degrees F. Place a 10-inch cast-iron skillet in the oven and let it heat up for 5 minutes.

2   While the pan is heating, combine the masa, garbanzo bean flour, baking powder, salt, oregano, thyme, olive oil, and maple syrup in a bowl and mix well.

3   Take the cast-iron pan out of the oven, being careful not to burn yourself. Add 1 Tbsp. of olive oil to the pan and spread evenly across the bottom and sides. Pour the batter into the pan and gently spread around by smoothly rocking the pan from side to side and end to end.

4   Bake the *farinata* in the oven for 10–12 minutes, or until the top is light golden brown. Let it cool for about 10 minutes before slicing and serving.

Island-Style Coconut Bacon

MAKES 3 CUPS

How do we begin to explain how mind-blowing this coconut bacon is? We are not sure there are words to describe it, but one taste and you'll see what we mean! The process for making this coconut bacon is simple and quick but demands attention. You'll need to stir it every five minutes for optimal results. Coconut bacon is so fun to have on hand to add pizzazz to your salad or to sprinkle on top of a baked potato with our scrumptious Cashew Cream Everything Sauce (page 198). Or, if you're like us, you might even eat it straight out of the jar. The coconut aminos and liquid smoke can be found in health-food stores. Also, remember to buy the wide unsweetened coconut flakes, as the smaller flakes will not work. This recipe is gluten free, soy free, and loaded with healthy fats. Five stars in our book!

3 Tbsp. coconut aminos

2 Tbsp. maple syrup

2 Tbsp. liquid smoke

1 tsp. paprika

¼ tsp. Himalayan pink salt

3 cups large unsweetened coconut flakes

1   Preheat the oven to 325 degrees F. Lightly oil a large baking sheet with extra-virgin coconut oil.

2   In a large bowl, mix together the coconut aminos, maple syrup, liquid smoke, paprika, and salt. Add the coconut flakes and stir until all the coconut is well covered.

3   Spread the coconut flakes on the oiled baking sheet. Bake for 20 minutes, stirring the coconut flakes every 5 minutes. (Reset the timer every 5 minutes to be safe.) Do not skip this step, or your coconut bacon will burn.

4   Remove the coconut flakes from the oven and let cool completely. Store in a glass jar or container in your pantry or on your countertop for up to two weeks.

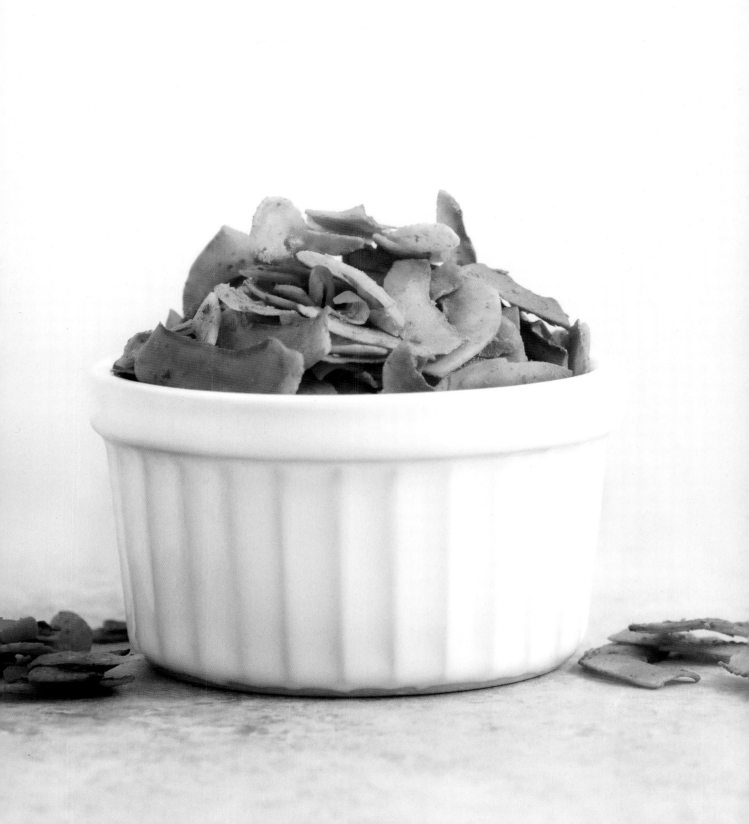

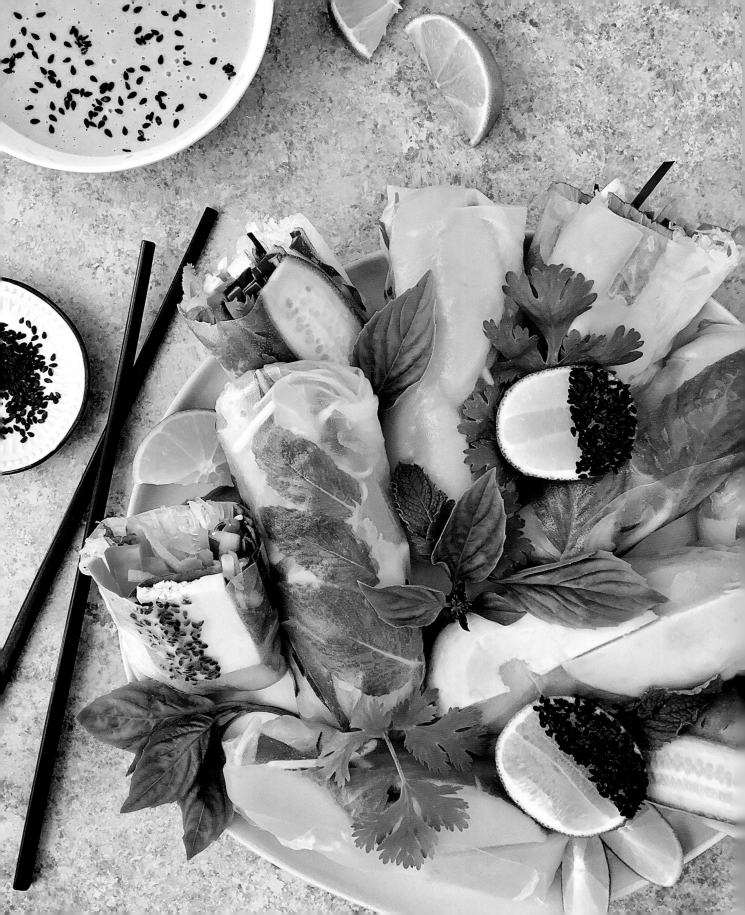

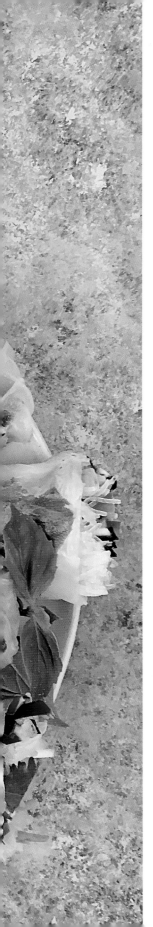

Summer Rolls with Thai Peanut Sauce

MAKES ABOUT 16 ROLLS

Summer Rolls are a fun and fresh finger food. They're versatile, too. Fill them with your favorite veggies, fruit, mung noodles, and tofu, and your taste buds will be bursting with delight. They do take a little bit of time to make, but they're worth the effort. Packed with healthy fats, protein, and fiber, these bite-size rolls satisfy and energize. Though they're a party favorite, they are just as delicious on a dinner plate and will keep the whole family at the table, asking for more. The Thai Peanut Sauce (page 190) is epic and pulls the entire dish together.

8 oz. mung noodles

1 carrot, julienned

1 red, orange, or yellow bell pepper, seeded and julienned

1 cucumber, peeled and julienned

1 cup julienned purple cabbage

½ block firm tofu, sliced into thin strips

1 mango, peeled, seeded, and sliced into thin strips

1 avocado, peeled, seeded, and sliced into thin strips

Handful of cilantro

Handful of Thai basil or mint, destemmed

16 sheets of round rice paper, about 9 inches in diameter (we use the brown rice papers, though the white rice papers are much more translucent and prettier for presentation)

Black sesame seeds

Thai Peanut Sauce (page 190)

▶

Summer Rolls with Thai Peanut Sauce *(cont.)*

1 In a medium pot, bring 4 cups of water to a boil. Add the noodles and turn off the heat, letting them cook for about 10 minutes. (Follow the directions on the package.) Once they are soft, drain them, rinse, and set aside.

2 Place the veggies, tofu, mango, avocado, and herbs in separate sections on a cutting board or individual bowls. Have fun with this part and choose colorful fruits and veggies and fresh herbs from the garden or farmers' market.

3 Fill a large bowl or a pie pan with warm water. Working with one piece of rice paper at a time, dunk the rice paper in the water and turn it from time to time until it softens, about 30 seconds.

4 Lay the softened rice paper sheet down on your work area. (We use a clean cutting board or large platter.) Place one strip of tofu and a small amount of noodles down first, then layer on your veggies, mango, and avocado, and top them off with a few sprigs of herbs and a sprinkle of black sesame seeds. Fold the bottom half over the filling, fold the sides in toward the middle, and roll up until the seam is tight and sealed. The tighter you can roll it, the better. If this seems confusing, refer to the photos on the rice paper packaging. But it's really quite simple and fun once you get the hang of it.

5 Serve the Summer Rolls on a large platter or plate with the Thai Peanut Sauce in a bowl on the side for dipping. The Summer Rolls can be stored in an airtight container overnight, but they taste best freshly made.

Eggless Egg Salad

MAKES ABOUT 4 CUPS

One of our son's favorites, this hearty Eggless Egg Salad fuels his energy for hours. It's nutritious and high in protein. Take this salad on a picnic or eat it for a quick snack. You can put it on an open-face sandwich with sliced avocado and sprouts or scoop it on top of your favorite greens. It's super good with crackers or pita, too!

2 blocks sprouted organic firm tofu

½ cup vegan mayonnaise, such as Vegenaise

⅓ cup nutritional yeast

½ cup diced celery

2 Tbsp. yellow mustard

1½ tsp. Spike seasoning

½ tsp. turmeric powder

½ tsp. Himalayan pink salt

1   Squeeze all of the liquid out of the tofu with a paper towel. In a medium-size bowl, mash the tofu with your hands until it is crumbly.

2   Add the vegan mayonnaise, nutritional yeast, diced celery, mustard, Spike, turmeric, and salt. Mix well.

3   Refrigerate in an airtight container for up to 1 week.

Picnic Potato Salad

SERVES 4

This is a perfect side dish. It works with all sorts of dishes and for all sorts of occasions, whether you're having a picnic, enjoying a simple dinner at home, or packing up a lunch to take to work. Roasting the potatoes instead of boiling them gives this classic dish a whole new twist. Our family unanimously votes for this roasted version every time we make potato salad. Of course, if you would like to boil them the traditional way, this recipe will still work. It's all a matter of taste.

8 cups of baby red potatoes, washed well and chopped in half

1 Tbsp. olive oil

¼ tsp. Himalayan pink salt, or more to taste

Pepper to taste

⅔ cup vegan mayonnaise, such as Vegenaise

½ cup finely chopped celery

½ cup sliced black olives

2 Tbsp. mustard

4 Tbsp. relish

4 Tbsp. finely chopped fresh dill

4 Tbsp. finely chopped fresh chives

1   Preheat the oven to 400 degrees F. Line a medium-size baking sheet with parchment paper.

2   In a large bowl, toss the potato halves with the olive oil and sprinkle with salt and pepper. Transfer to the baking sheet.

3   Roast the potatoes for about 40 minutes, tossing them halfway through. When they are cooked, let them cool for at least 20 minutes.

4   In a large bowl, mix together the vegan mayonnaise, celery, black olives, mustard, and relish.

5   Toss the cooled potatoes together with the dressing. Add the fresh dill and chives and season with salt and pepper to taste.

6   Serve warm or refrigerate for a cold potato salad.

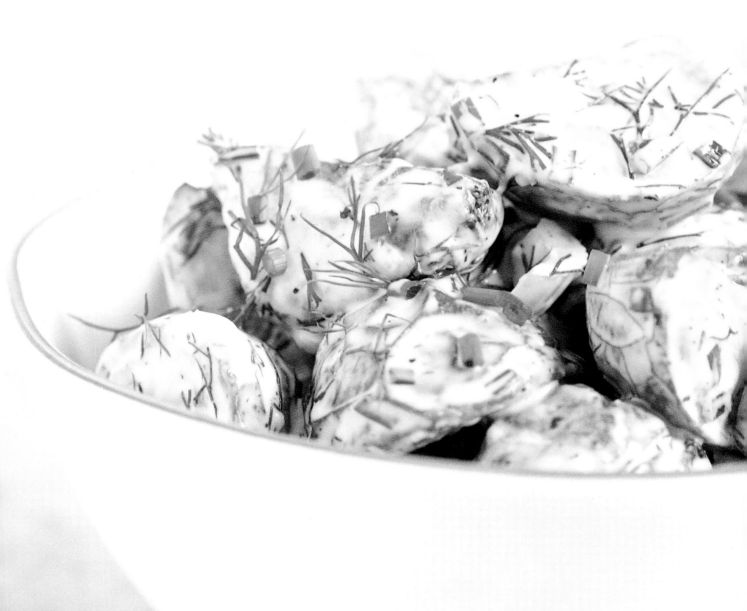

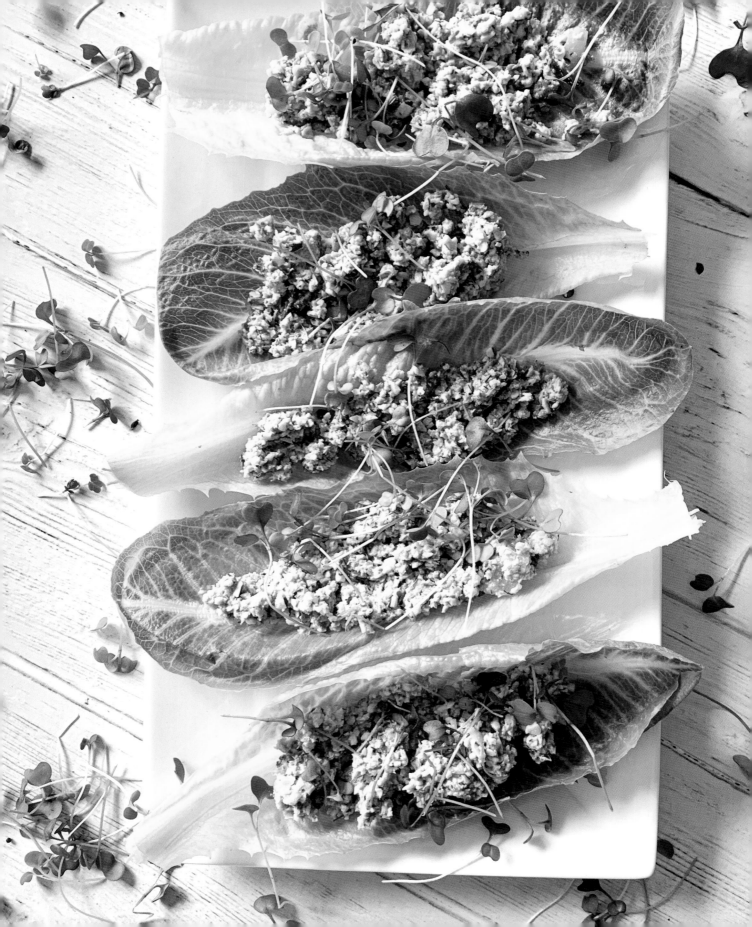

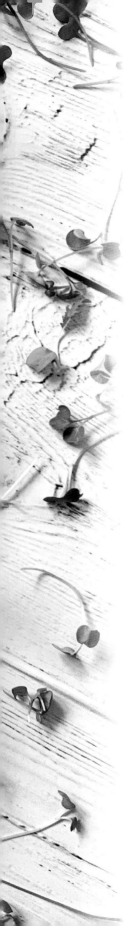

"Un" Tuna Salad

Save the dolphins with this classic plant-based sandwich spread. Made from sprouted nuts and seeds, this "Un" Tuna Salad is loaded with nutrition and energy-giving vitamins and minerals. The almonds and sunflower seeds are sprouted and raw, so they are "living" foods, which deliver all sorts of benefits that disappear with cooking. So while you are doing the right thing for the planet, you're also making a great choice for your body. This salad is bursting with vitamin E, copper, selenium, fiber, and antioxidants. Spread it on sandwich bread or on crackers or put a heaping spoonful on top of your favorite salad.

1 cup raw almonds

½ cup raw sunflower seeds

¼ cup water

2 Tbsp. lemon juice

2 sticks of celery, minced

2 Tbsp. minced red onion

2 Tbsp. minced fresh dill

2 Tbsp. nutritional yeast

1 tsp. tamari sauce

½ tsp. Spike seasoning

½ tsp. Himalayan pink salt

⅓ cup sweet pickle relish (optional)

1   Place the raw almonds and raw sunflower seeds in a bowl of water. The water should be at least 2 inches above the seeds. Soak for at least 8 hours or overnight. Drain and rinse.

2   Place the soaked almonds and sunflower seeds in a food processor and process into a paste. You may need to scrape down the sides a bit with a spatula.

3   Add all the remaining ingredients except the pickle relish to the food processor. Process until the mixture is chunky. (We just pulse it a few times.)

4   If using the pickle relish, stir it in by hand.

5   Store in an airtight container in the refrigerator for up to 5 days.

Autumn Roasted Veggies

SERVES 4

Roasted vegetables can be the best dish on the table or the worst. If they come out soggy and mushy, then they're ruined. The key is to spread the vegetables out on a baking sheet so that they aren't touching, which allows the vegetables to breathe and roast evenly. We like to create unique variations of roasted vegetables, stepping outside the mold of tradition. This recipe uses fennel root, carrots, radishes, parsnips, and a light balsamic sauce, topped with parsley and fennel fronds to give it extra color and depth. The fusion of these vegetables and the synergy between the sweet flavors of the roots and the tangy zest of the balsamic make for a dreamy combination. With a fresh twist like this, the vegetables are more exciting, more colorful, more fun, and even more scrumptious to eat.

3 cups ¼-inch-thick pieces of fennel root

8 small carrots, peeled

2 cups radish halves

1 cup inch-thick pieces of peeled parsnips

1 Tbsp. grape-seed oil

¼ tsp. Himalayan pink salt, or to taste

½ tsp. oregano

2 Tbsp. olive oil

2 tsp. balsamic vinegar

2 tsp. maple syrup

¼ cup minced parsley (garnish)

¼ cup fennel fronds (garnish)

1   Preheat the oven to 425 degrees F. Line two medium-size baking sheets with parchment paper.

2   Set the vegetables in a large bowl and cover them in 1 Tbsp. grape-seed oil, salt, and oregano. Mix until the vegetables are coated.

3   Transfer the veggies to the baking sheets, spreading them out evenly so they can cook properly. Roast in the oven for 25–30 minutes, or until they are light golden brown.

4   Whisk the 2 Tbsp. olive oil, balsamic vinegar, and maple syrup in a bowl for 1–2 minutes, until they emulsify.

5   Spoon the veggies onto a serving platter or individual plates, lightly drizzle over with the balsamic sauce, and serve right away. Garnish with parsley and fennel fronds.

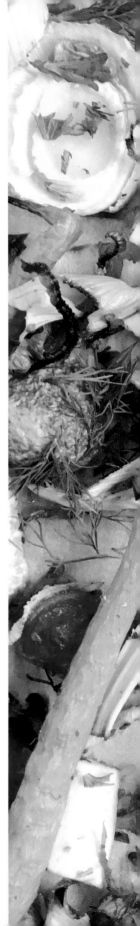

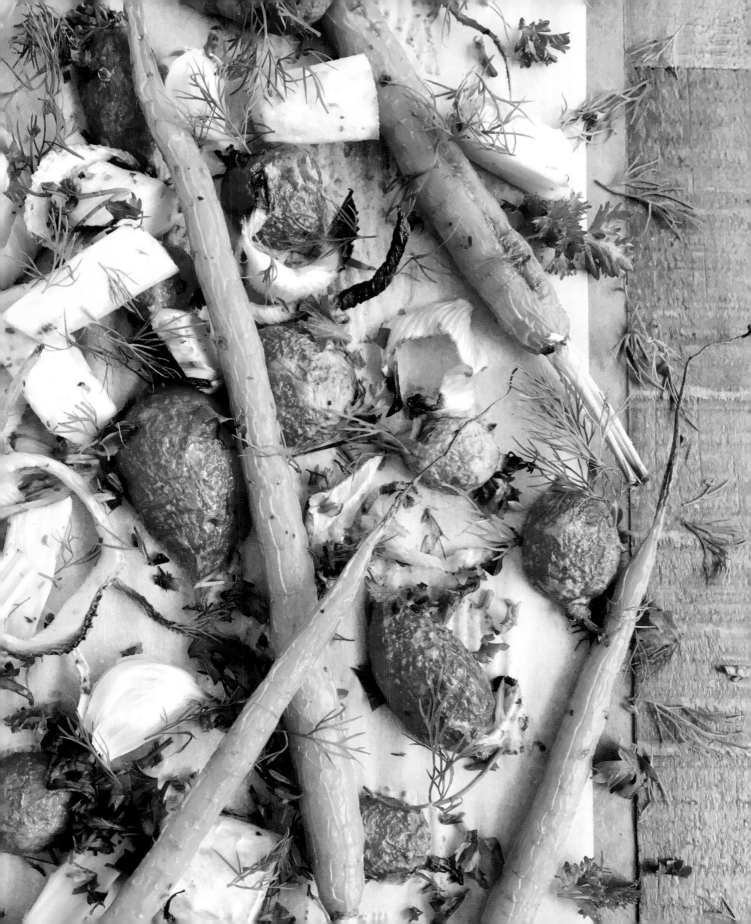

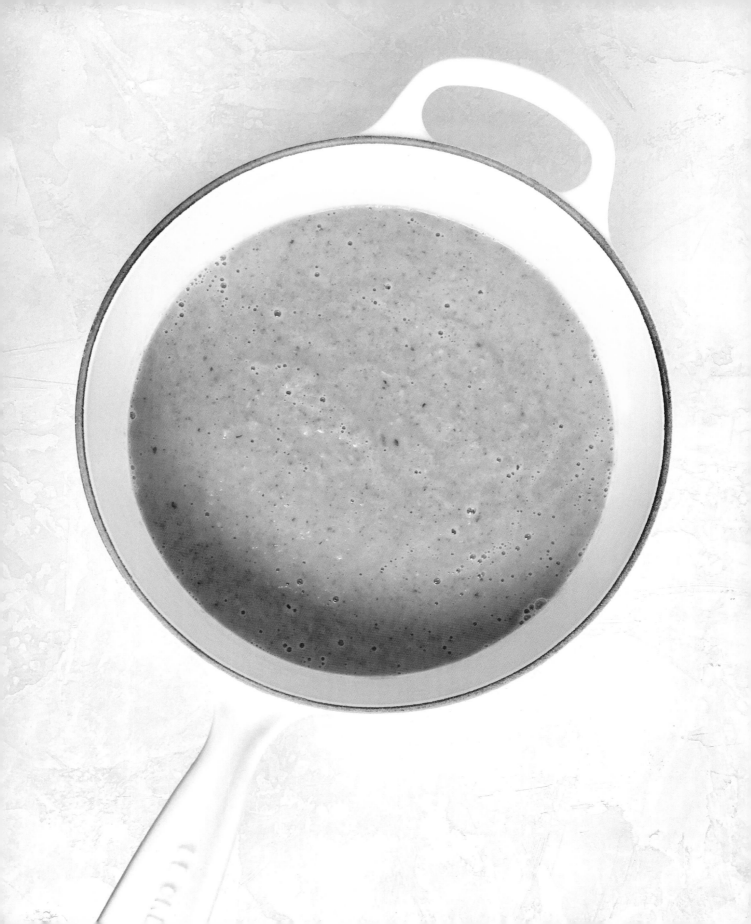

soups

Carrot Ginger Soup

Once the air becomes crisp and cool and the leaves start to change color, this is the perfect recipe to celebrate autumn. Carrot Ginger Soup will make you feel warm and cozy. You can make it as spicy or as mild as you like by adding more or less ginger. Rich in antioxidants and anti-inflammatory nutrients, this soup will keep you and your family healthy from the first days of fall all the way through winter and beyond. It is a great side dish for holiday season gatherings, too. It's simple to prepare but comes across as fancy and decadent. Try it out and see for yourself.

1 small onion, chopped (about 1 cup)

2 cloves garlic, peeled

2-inch piece of ginger root, peeled and finely chopped

3 Tbsp. olive oil

9–10 large organic carrots, roughly chopped (about 4 cups)

2 cups organic vegetable broth

1 tsp. Himalayan pink salt

Destemmed cilantro and/or croutons (garnish)

1 In a large pot over medium heat, sauté the onion, garlic, and ginger in the olive oil until tender.

2 Add the chopped carrots, broth, and salt to the pot. Bring to a boil, then reduce to a simmer, cover, and cook until the carrots are tender.

3 Take the pot off the burner and let the vegetables and broth cool. Pour about 2 cups of the mixture into a blender and blend on low speed until smooth. Pour that mixture into a medium-size bowl and continue blending the remaining vegetables and the broth until everything is blended. Add more broth if you want the soup to be a little thinner. (It will thicken up when you store it in the refrigerator.)

4 When all the soup is blended, pour back into the pot and heat until warm. Serve in bowls with cilantro and/or croutons for garnish. Add a drizzle of the Cashew Cream Everything Sauce (page 198) to make it extra special.

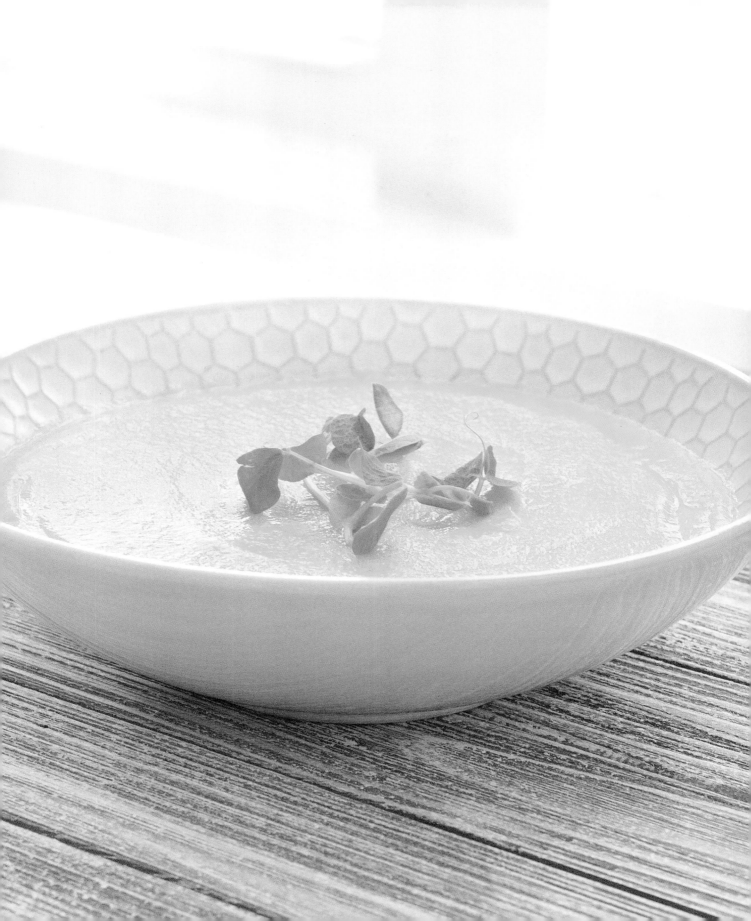

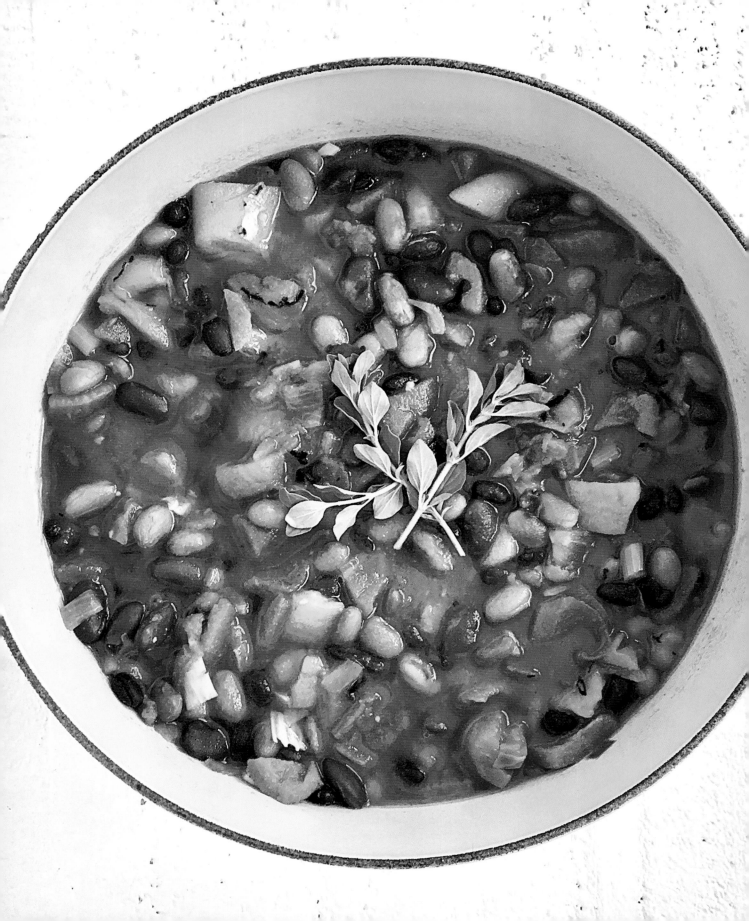

Hearty Vegan Chili

SERVES 6–8

Hearty, satisfying, and nutrient packed, this chili will leave you feeling full and energetic for hours. It is exploding with protein and fiber. This is the perfect dish to set on your table during a large party, particularly on a cold fall day. And even if it's a last-minute gathering, you'll be fine, because it takes only about 15 minutes to whip up. You'll have everyone talking about the medley of flavors in this dish. Serve it with avocado slices, destemmed or chopped cilantro, and a swirl of our Cashew Cream Everything Sauce (page 198). Makes great leftovers, too!

2 garlic cloves, peeled and minced

1 red onion, peeled and diced

2 Tbsp. olive oil

2 stalks celery, finely chopped

½ red bell pepper, seeded and finely chopped

1 jalapeño pepper, finely chopped (optional)

2 cups diced tomatoes, with their juice

1 cup water or vegetable broth

1 can pinto beans, drained and rinsed

1 can black beans, drained and rinsed

1 can kidney beans, drained and rinsed

1 Tbsp. cumin

1 Tbsp. chili powder (optional)

1 Tbsp. fresh or dried oregano

2 tsp. Himalayan pink salt

1 8-oz. jar roasted red or yellow bell peppers, diced (about 1 cup)

Toppings of choice (optional)

1 In a large pot over medium heat, sauté the minced garlic and diced onion in the olive oil for about 5 minutes, or until the onion is tender and translucent. Add celery, red peppers, and jalapeño and sauté for another 5 minutes.

2 Add tomatoes (with their juice) and the water or broth. Stir mixture well. Turn the heat up to medium-high and add the rinsed beans, spices, and roasted red or yellow bell peppers. Cook for about 10–15 minutes, until the chili has thickened.

3 Serve in bowls, topped with avocado slices, Cashew Cream Everything Sauce (page 198), and destemmed or chopped cilantro.

Bombay Red Lentil Soup

SERVES 6–8

The beauty of this dal (a term used in India for dried split lentils, peas, or beans) is that in just under 30 minutes, it'll fill your house with the aroma of all sorts of delicious spices and will make you feel like you are in India. From your first bite to the bottom of the bowl, this soup will nourish you. The lentils are filled with fiber and protein. This dish also packs in antioxidant elements and immune-boosting ingredients. A feel-good soup, it can be as mild or as spicy as you want. We love topping our bowls with fresh cilantro, scallions, and a dollop of our Cashew Cream Everything Sauce (page 198).

1 Tbsp. coconut oil

1 cup diced onion

1 garlic clove, peeled and minced

1 tsp. turmeric powder

1 tsp. cumin

⅛ tsp. cayenne (optional)

1 cup red lentils, washed and with the stones picked out

1 carrot, diced

4 cups vegetable broth

2 cups water

2 tsp. Himalayan pink salt

¼ tsp. pepper

2 Tbsp. lemon juice

1 cup baby spinach

½ cup diced tomatoes

Toppings of choice (optional)

1 Heat the coconut oil in a large soup pot over medium heat. Add the diced onion, minced garlic, turmeric, cumin, and cayenne (if using) and sauté until the spices are blended in and the onion is tender.

2 Add in the lentils, carrot, vegetable broth, water, salt, and pepper. Bring to a boil, then reduce to a simmer. Let simmer, uncovered, for about 20–30 minutes, or until the lentils fall apart.

3 Add lemon juice, spinach, and diced tomato just before serving. Let the spinach wilt and stir to mix it in.

4 Serve in bowls, topped with chopped cilantro, chopped scallions, and a swirl of our Cashew Cream Everything Sauce (page 198).

5 Store in an airtight container for up to 1 week.

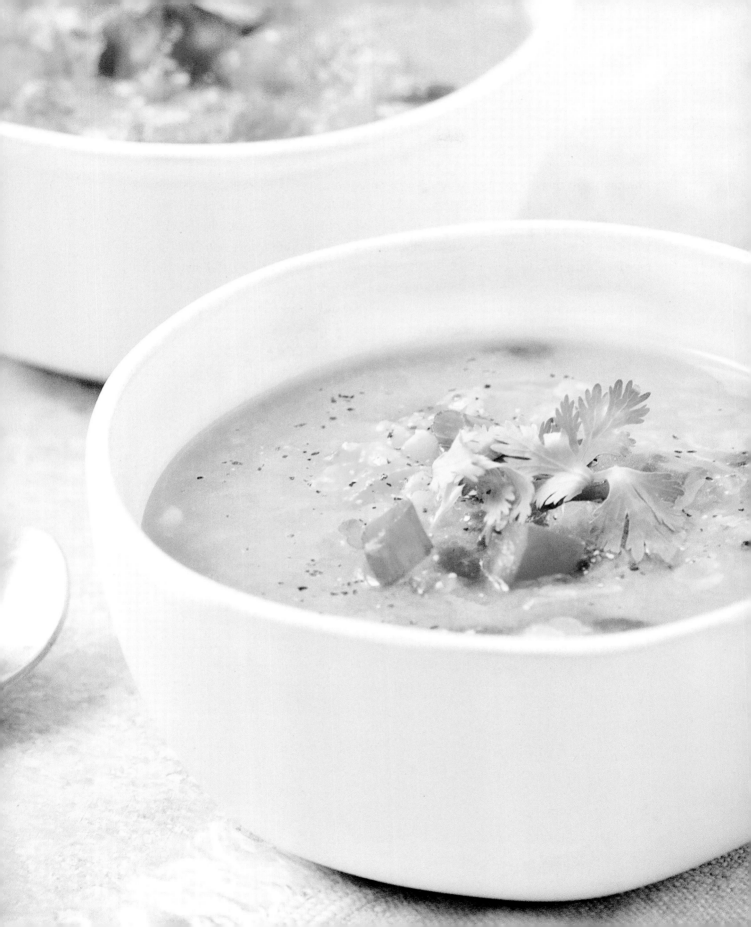

Miso Ramen Bowl

SERVES 4

Ramen is the archetypal Japanese street food. And miso is the healing, nutritious soup that has been used in the East, just like chicken noodle soup has been used in the West, to cure all ills, from colds to a lowered immune system. This recipe merges the two to form a powerful, well-balanced meal that dances on the tongue *and* fulfills our nutritional needs. While the recipe gives specific timing directions for adding the ingredients, you don't have to feel rushed when making this. Play around with the timing. Test the noodles as they boil; if they are slightly tender but not fully cooked, you know you have some time left and can add in the veggies.

3 Tbsp. miso paste

1 Tbsp. soy sauce

1 tsp. rice vinegar

1 tsp. sesame oil

2 Tbsp. plus 4 cups water

2 packs ramen noodles

1 cup broccoli, cut into small pieces

1 cup chopped shiitake mushrooms

1 cup spinach

1 cup chopped firm tofu

¼ cup minced scallions

½ cup nori (seaweed) strips, cut with scissors

Black sesame seeds (garnish)

1   Mix miso, soy sauce, rice vinegar, sesame oil, and 2 Tbsp. water in a small bowl and set aside.

2   Boil 4 cups of water and add ramen noodles, stirring occasionally.

3   Two minutes before the noodles are done, add broccoli and stir.

4   One minute before the noodles are done, add the shiitake mushrooms, spinach, tofu, scallions, and seaweed strips. Stir, then turn off heat.

5   Add the miso mixture and mix well. Pour into bowls, garnish with black sesame seeds, and serve right away.

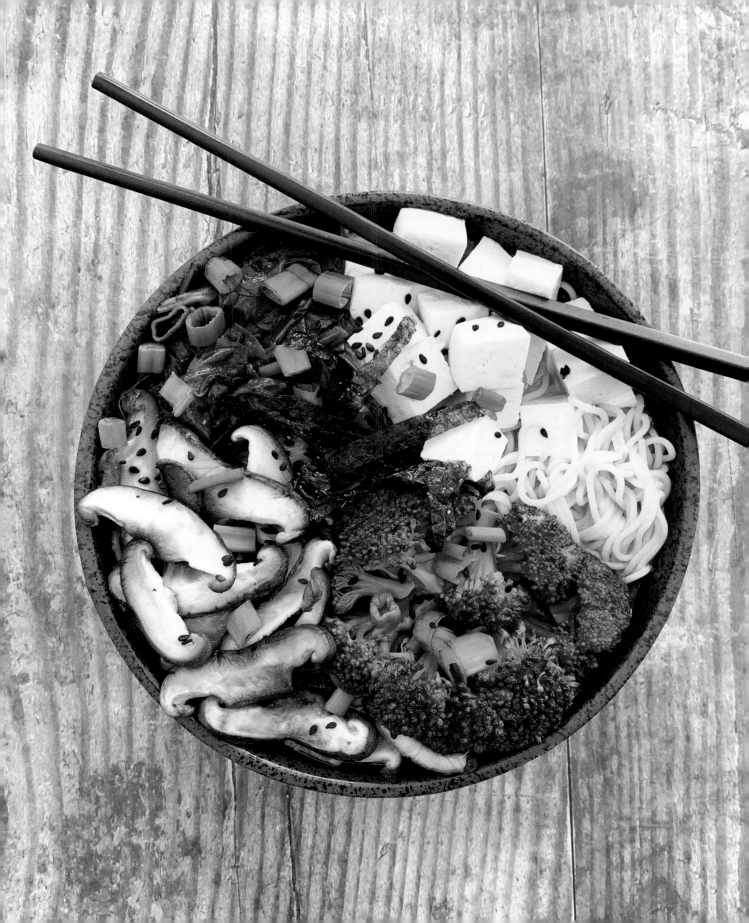

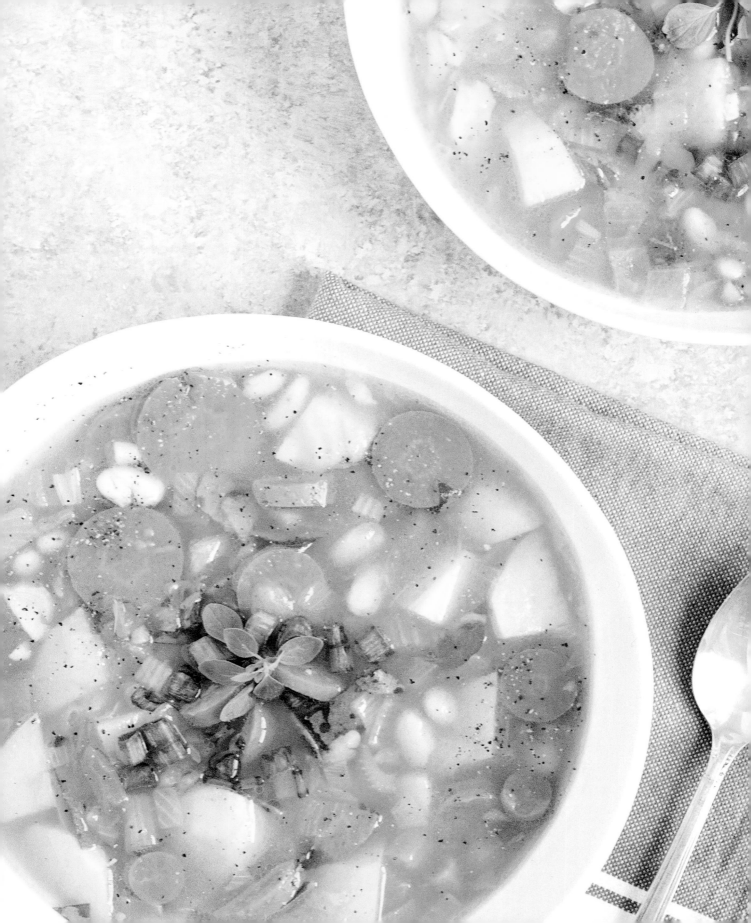

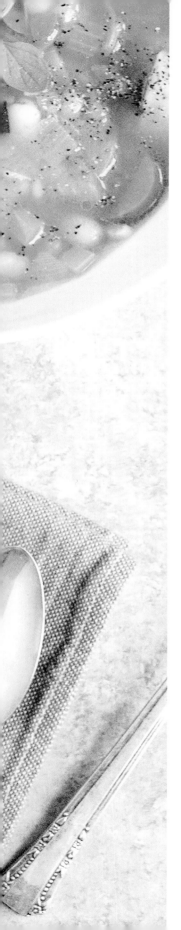

Cozy Winter White Bean Soup

SERVES 6–8

When it's cold outside, we turn to soups. A great soup can make you feel just as good as sitting by a wood stove on a wintry day. This Cozy Winter White Bean Soup will warm your heart and nourish your body. It'll sustain that warmth, too, filling you up and giving you energy to carry you right through the day. It's full of nutrients and protein. Pair it with some crusty whole-grain bread to make the perfect meal. Try making it for a holiday party — it's great for large groups.

2 Tbsp. olive oil

1 medium onion, diced (about 1 cup)

2 stalks celery, diced

3 cloves garlic, peeled and minced

2 cans white beans, drained and rinsed

2 medium potatoes, diced (about 2 cups)

2 large carrots, diced

1 Tbsp. finely chopped parsley

1 tsp. Himalayan pink salt

6 cups vegetable broth

1 cup water

Salt and pepper to taste

1   In a large soup pot, heat the olive oil over medium heat. Add onion, celery, and garlic and cook until the vegetables are tender.

2   Add the beans, potatoes, carrots, parsley, salt, 6 cups of broth, and 1 cup of water. Bring to a boil. Reduce the heat, cover, and simmer for about 1 hour. If necessary, add more water and salt and pepper to taste.

3   Store in an airtight container for up to 1 week.

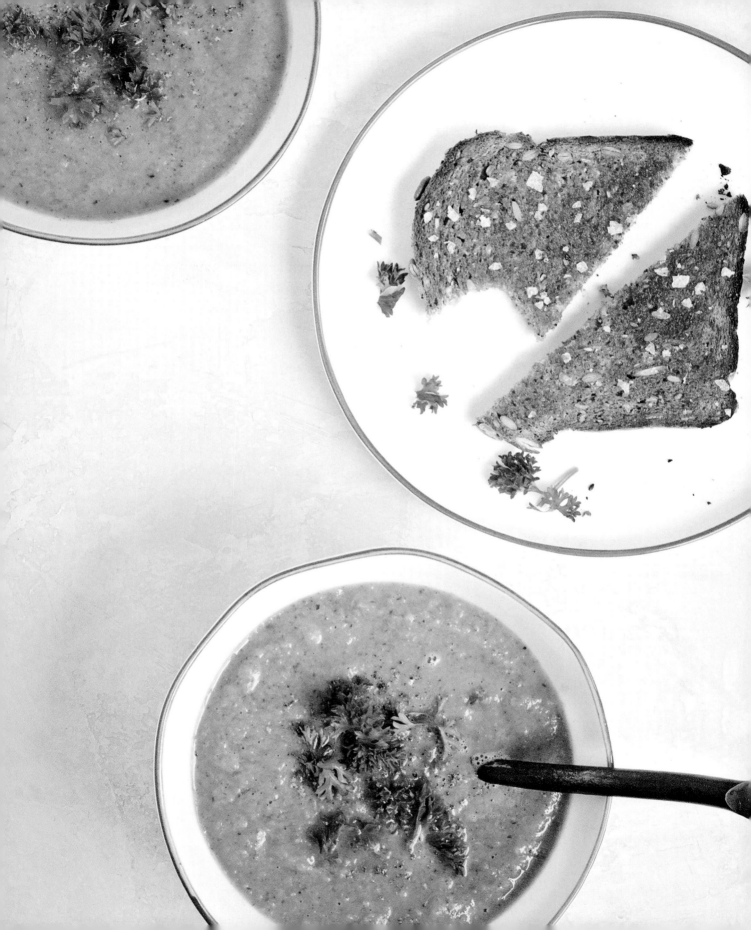

Green Soup

SERVES 6–8

This warm, savory soup is nourishing, clean, and full of Mother Nature's goodness. It's like a bowl full of heaven. Our Green Soup is light and packed with vitamins, minerals, and loads of fiber. Try a cup of this in the morning before you work out, particularly during those long winter months. It'll give you energy and comfort. Plus, you won't cut into your workout time—this takes only 30 minutes to prepare. Garnish with some of our Crunchy Croutons (page 144) or a little drizzle of our Cashew Cream Everything Sauce (page 198).

1 Tbsp. grape-seed oil

1 cup coarsely chopped onion

2 cups coarsely chopped celery

4 cups broccoli florets

1 medium-size zucchini, coarsely chopped

2 cups baby spinach

4 cups water

1 Tbsp. Himalayan pink salt

Pepper to taste

1 Heat the grape-seed oil in a large soup pot. Add the chopped onion and celery and sauté until the vegetables are slightly tender.

2 Add the broccoli, zucchini, spinach, water, salt, and pepper. Bring to a boil, then cover and simmer on low heat until all the vegetables are soft but not overcooked. They should still be vibrant green.

3 Turn the heat off. Scoop half of the soup mixture into a high-speed blender and blend until smooth. Pour into a bowl. Repeat with the remaining soup.

4 Pour all the blended soup back into the soup pot. Reheat to desired temperature and serve.

You can mix other vegetables into this recipe, too. Sometimes we substitute 2 cups cauliflower for half the broccoli. We also substitute kale or chard for the spinach when we feel like it. Use your imagination!

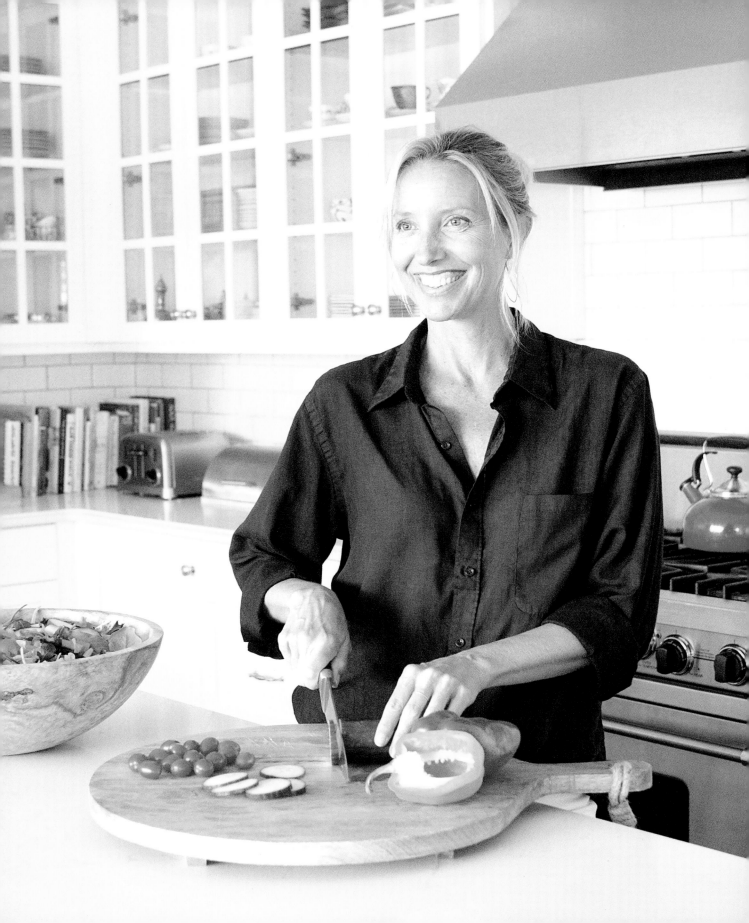

salads

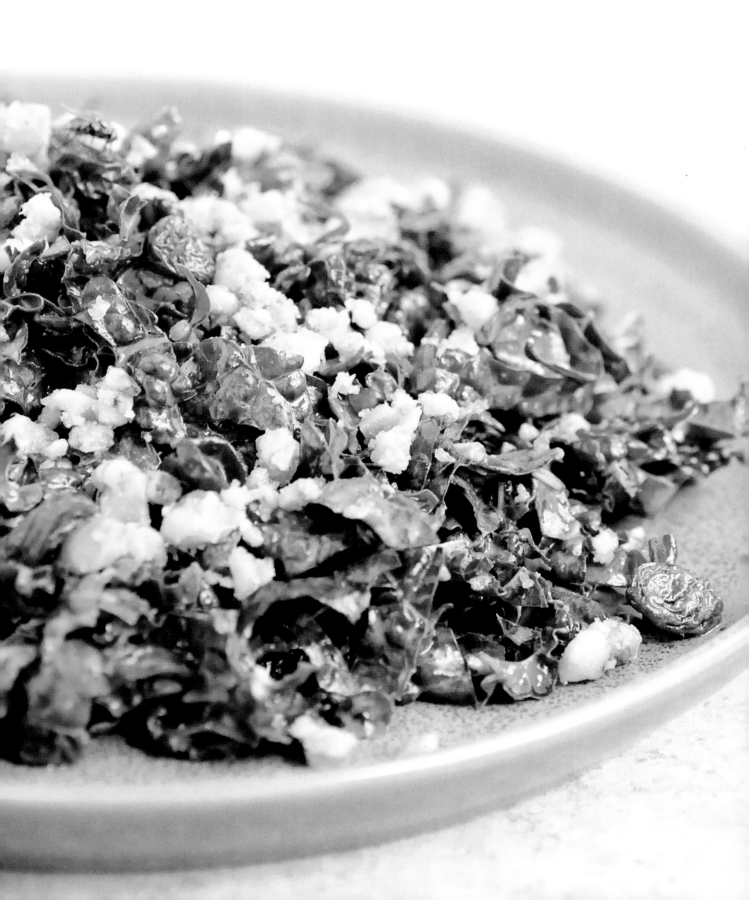

Our Favorite Kale Salad

SERVES 4–6

Kale is a powerhouse ingredient. It delivers loads of fiber, vitamin K, vitamin C, minerals, and antioxidants. This simple salad is a breeze to make, but the complex flavors will impress your friends and family. There's a sweet and salty duality in this dish that cuts the bitterness of the kale. This is a salad we always set on the table when we're hosting a dinner party or a big gathering. We switch the raisins to cranberries during the holiday season. It looks so pretty with those holiday colors of evergreen and deep red. Pair it with our Carrot Ginger Soup (page 114). We're confident this will become one of your favorite salads, too!

For the dressing

1 clove garlic, peeled

¼ cup olive oil

3 Tbsp. lemon juice

1 Tbsp. tahini

⅛ tsp. Himalayan pink salt

⅛ tsp. black pepper

1 Place the garlic in a mini food processor and mince.

2 Add the olive oil, lemon juice, tahini, salt, and black pepper and process until smooth and creamy. Set aside until the salad is ready.

For the Walnut Parmesan Cheese

½ cup raw walnuts

1 Tbsp. olive oil

1 Tbsp. nutritional yeast

⅛ tsp. Himalayan pink salt

1 Place the walnuts into a mini food processor and pulse until the nuts are reduced to small, rice-size bits.

2 Add the olive oil, nutritional yeast, and salt. Pulse again until the mixture looks like Parmesan cheese. Set aside until the salad is ready.

▶

Our Favorite Kale Salad *(cont.)*

For the salad

2 heads of dinosaur kale
(the dark, leafy one)

Olive oil (for drizzling)

¼ cup raisins, soaked in
water for about 5 minutes

1 Rinse the kale very thoroughly, pat the leaves dry, and destem them. Stack the leaves about five to six high and and cut them into very thin strips. Repeat with the remaining leaves.

2 Transfer the kale to a salad bowl. Drizzle with the olive oil. Massage the kale with your hands to soften it and help it absorb the oil.

3 Add the soaked raisins and toss together.

4 Toss the entire batch of Walnut Parmesan Cheese into the salad. Serve with as much dressing as you prefer.

You can easily double the Walnut Parmesan Cheese recipe, store the extra in an airtight container or mason jar in the fridge, and use often. For the salad, prepping the kale the day before can speed up the process.

Mexican Chop Salad

SERVES 4–6

This wonderful summer salad is full of vibrant colors and flavors that will brighten up any day. We love Mexican food in our house, so you'll find this on our table a lot, right beside our Holy Mole Guacamole! (page 89) and our Mango Salsa (page 199). Our son, Kanai, would eat beans every day of the week if he could. This dish is a fun and different way for him to enjoy his favorite protein; it's not the typical taco. Plus it delivers all of those hydrating fresh vegetables, and that makes a mom and dad smile from ear to ear. Try mixing the ranch dressing with a little salsa for even more flavor (it also makes a great dip for chips). There are no rules when it comes to taco salad, so have fun and be creative!

For the salad

4 cups chopped romaine

¾ cup chopped tomatoes

¾ cup corn (roasted is really good, but not necessary)

¾ cup chopped bell pepper

½ cup chopped cucumber

½ avocado, peeled, pitted, and diced

1 cup cooked black beans

½ cup chopped cilantro or more (we love cilantro, so we double this!)

¼ cup chopped scallion greens

For the ranch dressing

1 cup vegan mayonnaise, such as Vegenaise

¼ cup unsweetened nondairy milk

1½ tsp. apple cider vinegar

1 tsp. garlic powder

1 tsp. dried dill

1 tsp. dried parsley

1 tsp. onion powder

½ tsp. Himalayan pink salt

Pinch of pepper, to taste

▶

Mexican Chop Salad (*cont.*)

1 Combine the romaine, tomatoes, corn, bell
peppers, cucumber, and avocado in a large
salad bowl and toss together. Add the beans
and toss again.

2 In a mason jar, place all the ingredients for
the dressing, put on the lid, and shake until
blended. If you would like your dressing
thicker, refrigerate overnight.

3 Toss the salad with the dressing, coating the
vegetables to your desired level. Sprinkle on
the cilantro and scallions and serve.

*We like to crush up tortilla chips
to use as croutons.*

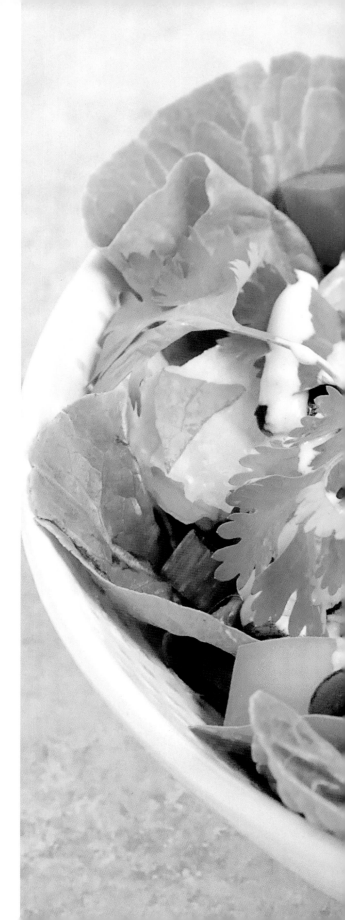

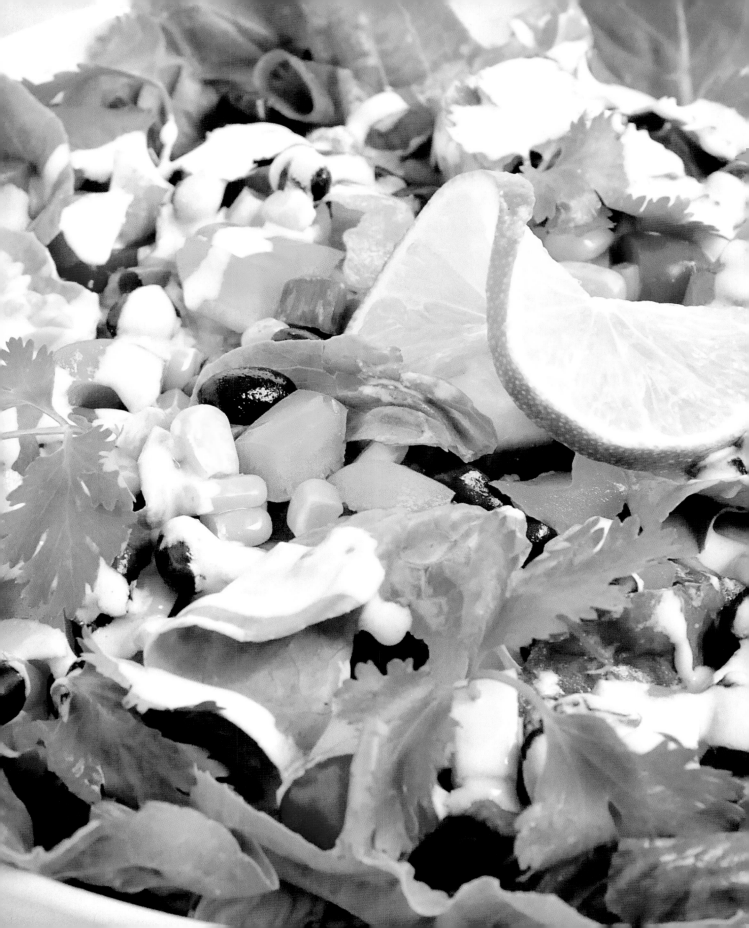

Coconut Ceviche

SERVES 4–6

When I think of perfect summer salads, Coconut Ceviche is at the top of the list. It's refreshing, colorful, nourishing, and filling. Loaded with healthy fats and fiber from the coconut meat and avocado, just one small bowl will leave you feeling completely satisfied. It takes a bit of effort to open the coconuts and scoop out the meat, but it's well worth it. The tomatoes and citrus provide high doses of vitamin C, as well as loads of antioxidants. Cilantro, one of our favorite herbs ever, has a citrusy flavor that tops this dish off perfectly. Studies have shown that cilantro has a detoxifying effect on the blood. I like to add fresh or frozen mango to this dish. The mango takes it to the next level, particularly on a hot summer day. Serve Coconut Ceviche on avocado halves; scoop it up with tortilla chips, like a salsa; or just simply eat as is.

3 young coconuts

¼ cup lemon juice

¼ cup lime juice

1 cup chopped tomatoes

¼ cup diced red onion

½ tsp. Himalayan pink salt, or to taste

½ cup chopped cilantro

1 avocado, peeled, pitted, and cubed

½ cup fresh or frozen mango cubes (optional, but oh so good!)

1 To open the coconuts: Place a coconut on its side. Shave the husks off the top point with a very sharp knife. Whack the sharp edge of the knife around the top of the coconut until you form a circle. Pry it open with a butter knife and pour the coconut water into a glass or jar; it is the sweetest water you will ever taste and is high in electrolytes, so be sure to keep it for drinking.

2 With a spoon, scoop the young coconut meat out of the shells and rinse well. Cut the coconut meat into small squares and place in a bowl.

3 Add in the lemon and lime juices and mix well.

4 Toss in the chopped tomatoes, diced red onion, and salt.

5 Cover and chill until serving time. Just before serving, toss in cilantro, avocado, and mango cubes. This salad will help you beat the heat!

For easy-to-follow visuals on opening a coconut, see the tutorial video "How to Open a Coconut" on Victoria's The Yoga Plate YouTube channel.

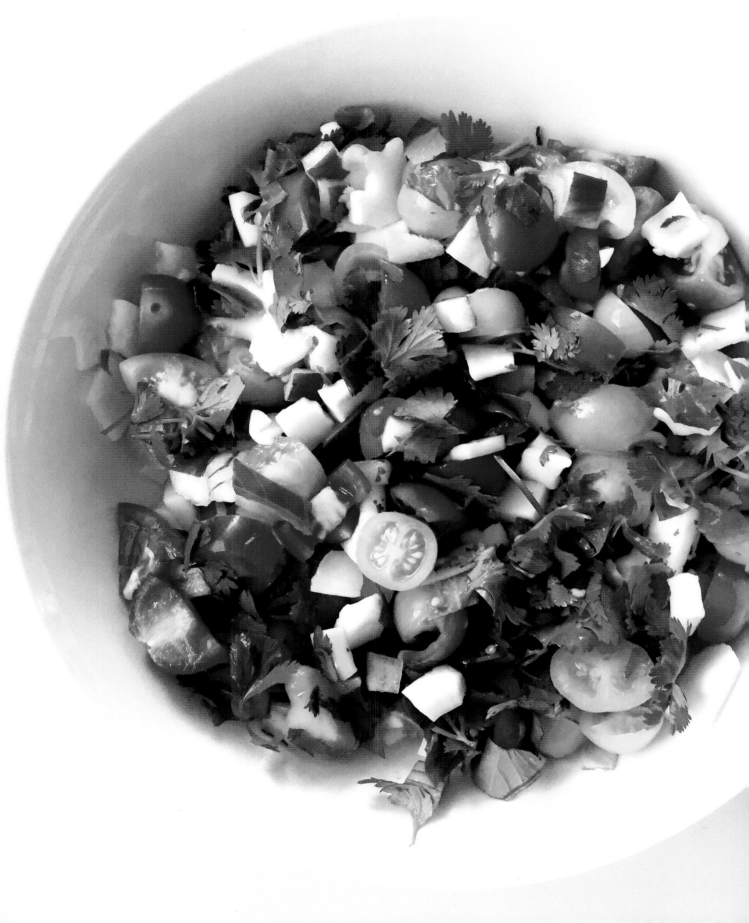

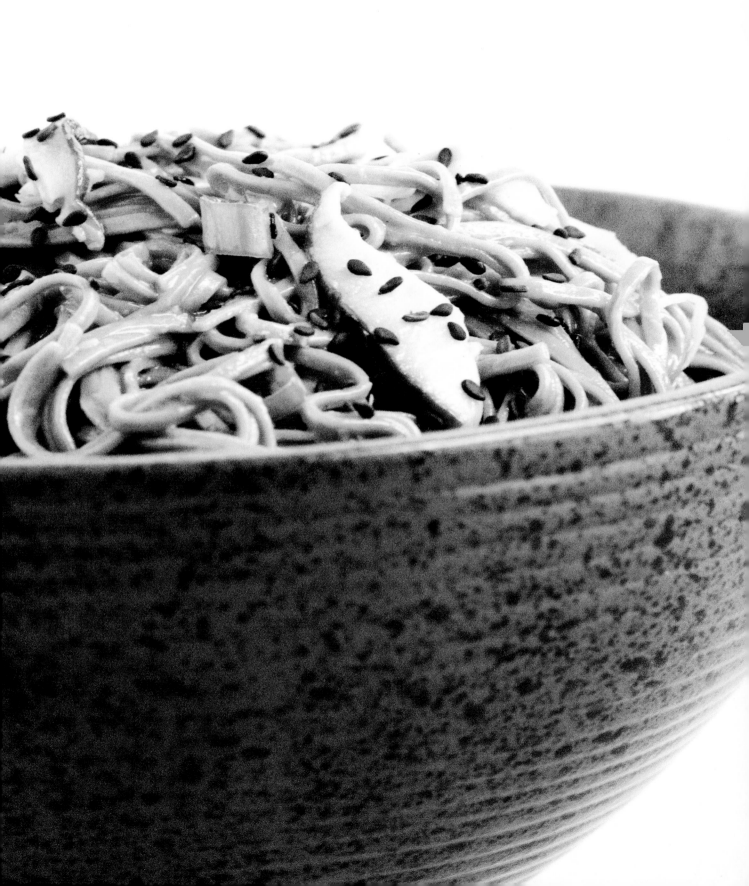

Tokyo Soba

If you swing by our house just about any night of the week, you'll catch the aroma of Japanese and Thai ingredients wafting from our kitchen. They're some of our favorite Asian food cooking styles. We count this Tokyo Soba as one of those household staples. It is sweet, tangy, and a little spicy, with a kick from the ginger dressing. The flavors in this dish are balanced, so that none of them eclipse the others. It's like a symphony on your palate.

1 9.5-oz package of buckwheat soba noodles

1 Tbsp. grape-seed oil

¼ cup finely chopped onion

1½ cups sliced shiitake mushrooms

¼ tsp. Himalayan pink salt

½ cup edamame beans, out of the pod

2 cups cabbage, chopped

½ tsp. sesame oil

¼ cup scallions

Miso Ginger Dressing (page 201)

1 tsp. black sesame seeds (garnish)

1   Cook the buckwheat soba according to the package instructions.

2   When the soba is done, drain it in a strainer, then pour ice water over it. This will prevent the soba from becoming mushy. Set the cool soba aside.

3   Heat the grape-seed oil in a large skillet. Toss in the onions and sauté for 2–3 minutes, or until they are tender. Add mushrooms and salt, sauté for another 2–3 minutes, then add edamame and cabbage and sauté for about 2 minutes more, until the cabbage is wilted and soggy.

4   Turn the heat off and stir in sesame oil for flavor. Transfer the veggies to a bowl to cool off.

5   In a large bowl combine the soba, veggies, and scallions. Douse the salad with the Miso Ginger Dressing and a little sprinkle of black sesame seeds.

Asian Kale Quinoa Salad

SERVES 4

This salad is one of our household staples. It takes only about 30 minutes from start to finish, and it is a crowd pleaser. Quinoa is not only gluten free, it is also a superfood, loaded with protein, fiber, magnesium, and iron. Plus, the seaweed is light and refreshing, yet extremely nourishing—though sometimes we'll omit the seaweed, depending on whom we are serving it to. And there are still plenty of healthy ingredients to enjoy. Kale is a powerhouse, filled with vitamin C, vitamin K, vitamin A, fiber, manganese, and copper. Avocado has healthy fats, and lemon is very cleansing. It's a hit in our house.

1 cup dry quinoa

2 cups water

1 cup (or more) kale, destemmed and ripped into small pieces

¼ cup olive oil

¼ cup nori (seaweed), cut into small pieces with scissors

2 small cucumbers, diced

1 avocado, peeled, pitted, and cubed

1 tsp. black sesame seeds

Juice from ½ lemon

½ tsp. garlic salt

½ tsp. Himalayan pink salt

1 Combine the quinoa and water in a small pot and bring to a boil. Cover, reduce heat to low, and cook for 20 minutes. Remove from burner and let cool.

2 After the quinoa has cooled a bit, scoop it into a large bowl. Add the kale, olive oil, nori, cucumbers, avocado, black sesame seeds, lemon juice, garlic salt, and salt. Toss together well and serve. It's that simple!

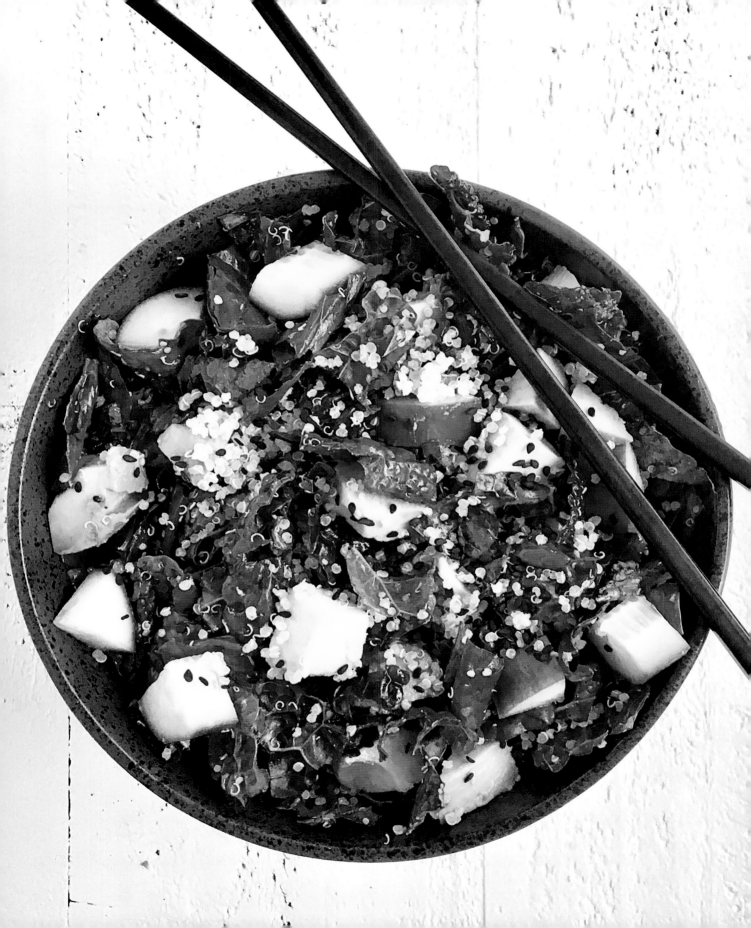

Summer Zucchini Salad

SERVES 4–6

Take your palate on a summer trip to Italy with this light, refreshing, colorful zucchini salad. The zucchini noodles can be prepared the day before for a quick on-the-go assembly. We love making this salad for our friends and family. It's perfect for a garden party or an afternoon picnic. Filled with wholesome nutrients and mouthwatering flavors, this is a must try for all!

2 medium-size zucchini

2 Tbsp. extra-virgin olive oil

Salt to taste

1 fresh heirloom tomato or 1 cup of baby tomatoes

½ cup chopped fresh basil

2 Tbsp. Cashew Parmesan Cheese (page 200)

1 Bring the zucchini to room temperature. Pass the zucchini through a spiral slicer and place the resulting noodles into a large bowl. Add the olive oil and salt and let the noodles soften for about 10–15 minutes.

2 Cut the heirloom tomato into small pieces or the baby tomatoes in half. Toss into the zucchini noodles.

3 Add the chopped basil and top off with Cashew Parmesan Cheese.

If you do not own a spiralizer, you can use a vegetable peeler to make long, thin noodles out of the zucchini.

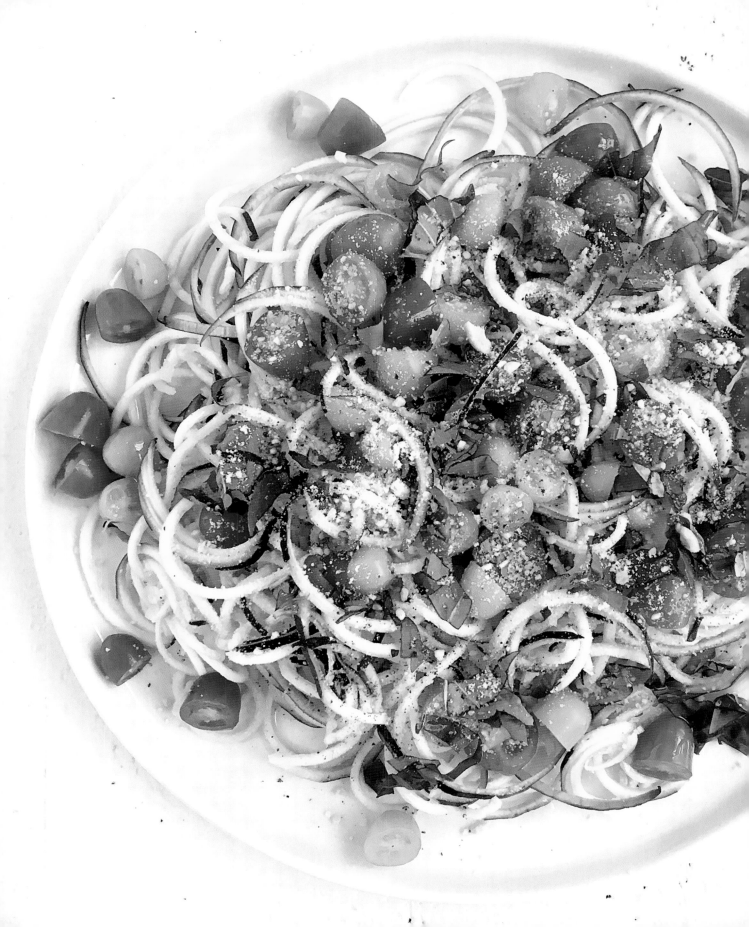

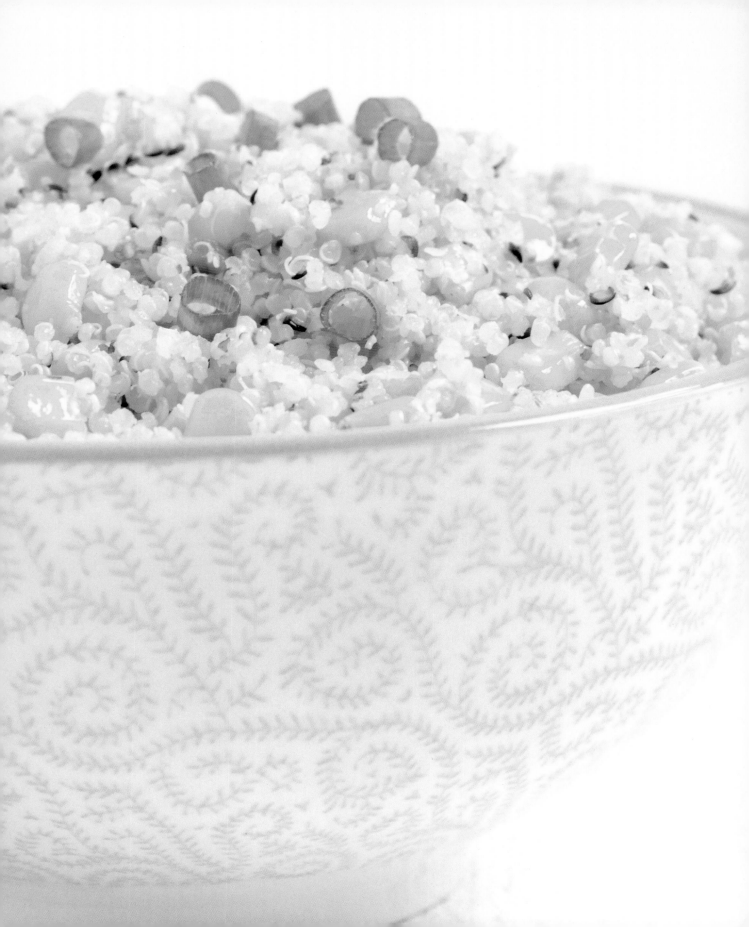

Refreshing Summer Quinoa Salad

SERVES 6–8

On a sweltering day, the best dishes are ones that somehow make you feel lighter. Fluffy, heart healthy, and delicious, this quinoa dish is the perfect balm during the hottest months of the year. It is loaded with healthy omegas, fiber, antioxidants, and healthy fats. It'll become a family favorite in no time. You can store it in the fridge to pull out for a quick snack between meals or serve it with a green salad or on top of our Stuffed Mexican Sweet Potato (page 173) for a delightful midsummer main course.

1 cup dry quinoa

2 cups water

1 Tbsp. coconut oil

1 garlic clove, peeled and minced

2 cups organic corn

2 scallions, thinly sliced

½ tsp. Himalayan pink salt

½ cup hemp seeds

1 Tbsp. chia seeds

Juice from ½ lemon

Pepper to taste

1 Place the quinoa and water in a small pot and bring to a boil. Cover and simmer on low heat for 20 minutes. Remove from the burner and let the quinoa cool.

2 Heat coconut oil in a sauté pan over medium heat. Add the garlic, corn, scallions, and salt and sauté for 3–4 minutes.

3 Transfer the cooked quinoa to a large bowl. Add in the sautéed corn mixture, hemp seeds, chia seeds, and lemon juice and toss together. Add the pepper and more salt to taste, tossing again. Serve warm or cold.

4 Store in an airtight container for up to 10 days.

Creamy Caesar Salad with Crunchy Croutons

SERVES 4–6

This is a delicious, creamy vegan Caesar salad that will dazzle your friends. We make extra croutons because the kids will devour every last one. (We actually fight over the croutons. True story!) This salad can be made the classic way, or if you want to spruce it up a bit, you can add some hearty kale to the mix. We love to make this on our pizza night; pizza and this Caesar make a perfect pair. If you are cooking for friends, you can cut down on prep time by making the Caesar dressing and the Cashew Parmesan Cheese (page 200) the day before.

For the Crunchy Croutons

6 slices whole-grain bread, cubed

2 Tbsp. olive oil

Sprinkle of garlic powder

Sprinkle of Himalayan pink salt

For the salad

2 small heads of romaine
(about 8–10 cups)

Cashew Parmesan Cheese (page 200)

For the dressing

½ cup cashews, soaked for 1 hour

¼ cup water

1 garlic clove, peeled

1½ tsp. capers, with juice

¼ cup olive oil

1 Tbsp. lemon juice

1 tsp. tamari or Bragg's
liquid aminos

⅛ tsp. Himalayan pink salt

1 tsp. Dijon mustard

Pinch of black pepper, to taste

1   Preheat the oven to 350 degrees F. Line a medium-size baking sheet with parchment paper.

2   In a medium bowl, toss the cubed bread chunks with the olive oil, garlic powder, and a sprinkle of salt.

3   Spread evenly on the baking sheet and bake for 15 minutes. Then flip the croutons over and bake for another 5 minutes. Take out of the oven to cool.

4   While the croutons are baking, place all ingredients for the dressing in a food processor or high-speed blender. Blitz until the dressing is smooth and creamy.

5   Rinse the romaine thoroughly and pat dry with a paper towel or dry with a salad spinner. Chop or tear the lettuce into bite-size pieces. Place in a large salad bowl.

6   Pour the dressing on the romaine and toss it until it's fully coated. Sprinkle Cashew Parmesan Cheese on top, toss on the Crunchy Croutons, and serve.

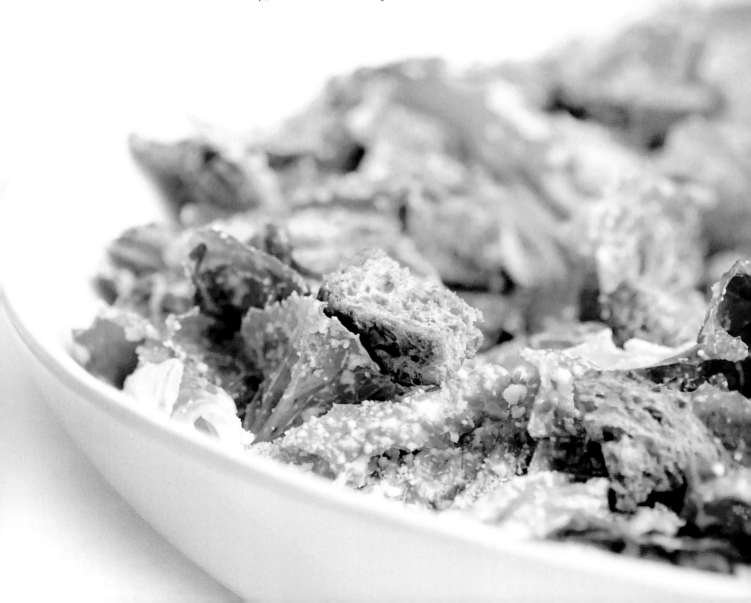

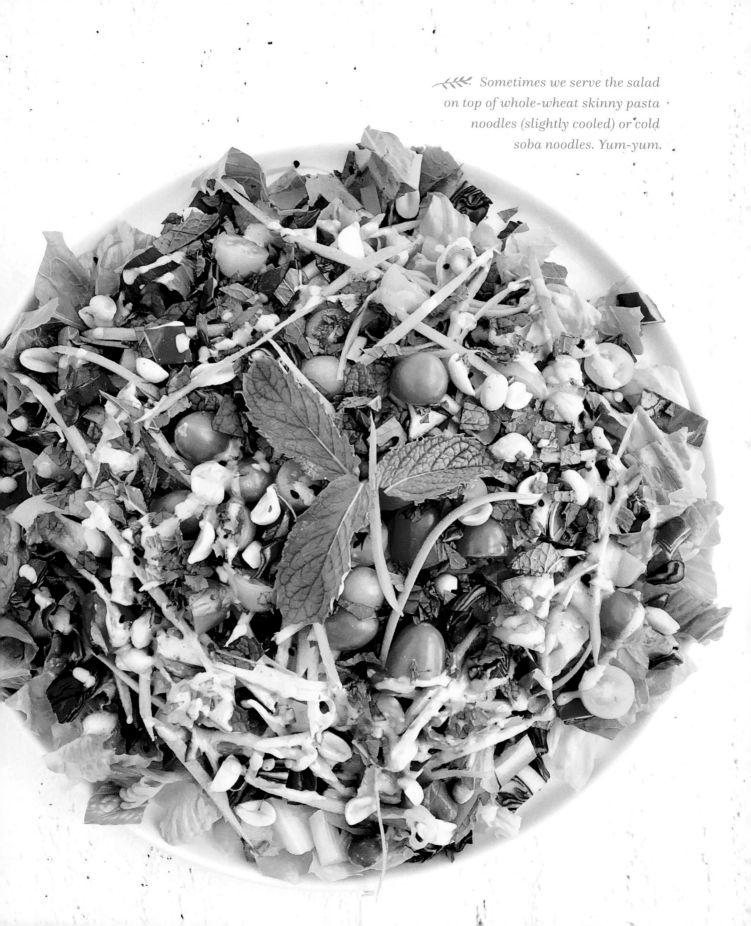

Sometimes we serve the salad on top of whole-wheat skinny pasta noodles (slightly cooled) or cold soba noodles. Yum-yum.

Crunchy Thai Salad

Colorful and bursting with flavors, this Thai salad isn't just something to serve at a gathering. It's part of the festivities! It's crunchy, hydrating, and loaded with fiber, not to mention heaps of vitamins and minerals. If you don't have a julienne tool, you can just chop the veggies into thin slices. And if you don't have time to make our Simple Peanut Dressing, simply replace it with your favorite store-bought version. However, we do have to warn you that homemade always tastes best! Make the salad dressing earlier in the day to save on time when you're getting ready to eat.

For the Simple Peanut Dressing

½ cup peanut or almond butter

¼ cup maple syrup

¼ cup rice wine vinegar

¼ cup sesame oil

3 Tbsp. soy sauce or tamari

2 Tbsp. lime juice

½ tsp. ginger powder

½ tsp. garlic powder

For the salad

½ cup chopped purple cabbage

1 tomato, chopped

1 cucumber, julienned

1 small red, yellow, or orange bell pepper, seeded and julienned

1 small carrot, julienned

1 large handful fresh cilantro, chopped (we use the entire bunch, but we love cilantro)

1 small handful fresh mint leaves, chopped

⅓ cup peanuts or raw cashews

½ cup cubed baked tofu (optional)

Salt to taste

6–8 romaine leaves, chopped

1   Pour all the Simple Peanut Dressing ingredients into a blender and process until smooth. If you want a thinner consistency, add 1 Tbsp. water at a time to thin out the dressing.

2   Place all the salad ingredients except the romaine into a large salad bowl. Toss with the peanut dressing.

3   Arrange a bed of romaine leaves on a platter, transfer the dressed salad onto the romaine, and serve.

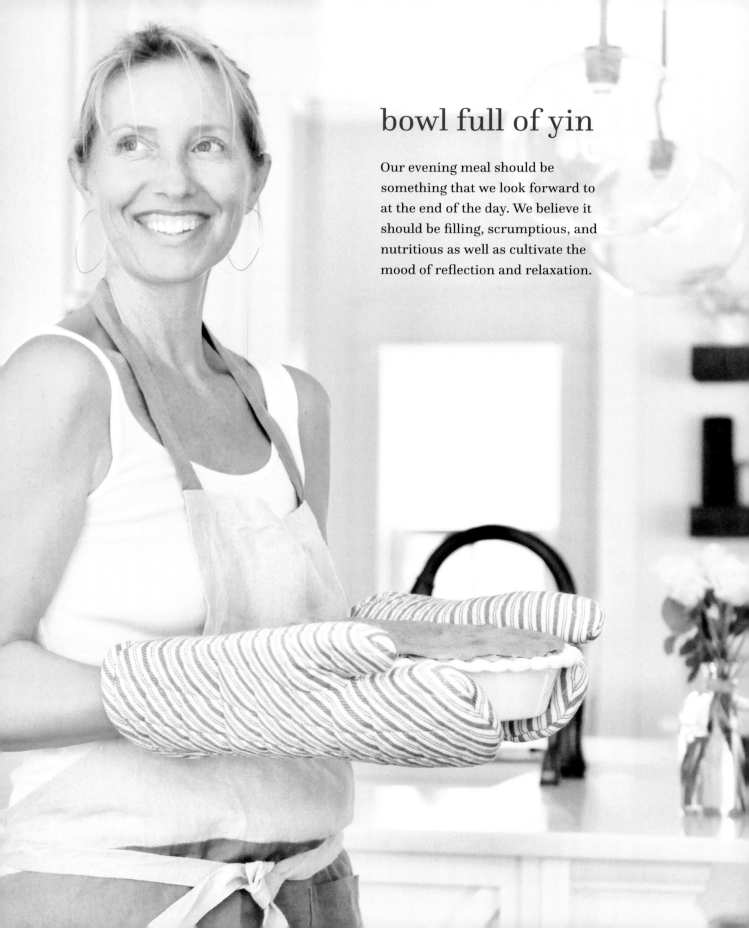

bowl full of yin

Our evening meal should be something that we look forward to at the end of the day. We believe it should be filling, scrumptious, and nutritious as well as cultivate the mood of reflection and relaxation.

entrées

The Monk Bowl

In our house we have a running joke that Victoria could live off of salad, brown rice, and lentils. We call her diet "monk food" because she is so simple in her food habits and she loves to eat clean, basic meals. This recipe is one of Victoria's all-time favorites, as it is simple and very satisfying. We play with many variations on cooking lentils in our house because we love the way lentils make our bodies feel. The Monk Bowl is super high in protein, fiber, and minerals that boost your energy and fuel your body as well as being easy to digest.

2 cups dry lentils

6 cups water

¼ cup lemon juice

¼ cup olive oil

½ tsp. paprika

½ tsp. finely chopped garlic

1 tsp. cumin

¼ cup finely chopped parsley

½ Tbsp. finely chopped chives

1¼ tsp. Himalayan pink salt

1   Rinse the lentils and pick out any stones. Place them in a large pot with the water. Bring to a boil, then turn the heat down to low and cover. Let the lentils simmer for 20 minutes, or until fully cooked.

2   Drain the lentils in a strainer and give them a light rinse with fresh water. Set them aside.

3   To make the marinade, place the rest of the ingredients in bowl and mix together well.

4   Pour the marinade over the cooked lentils and stir well. Serve over brown rice.

The best sauce for the Monk Bowl is the Magic Tahini Sauce (page 189), as its slightly bitter, sour taste complements the hearty flavor of the lentils and rice.

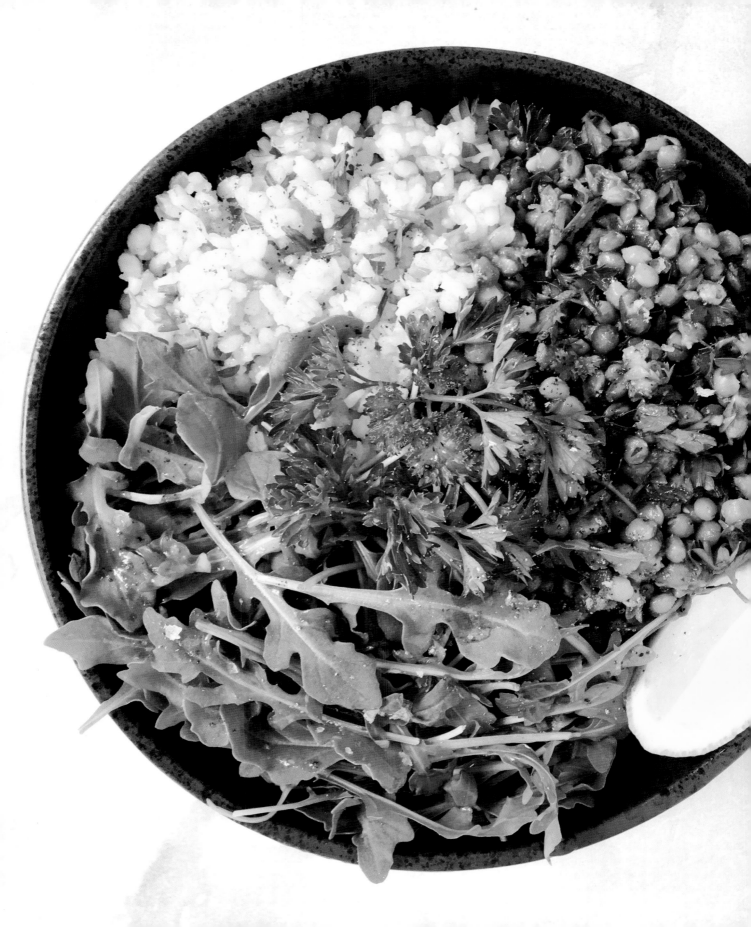

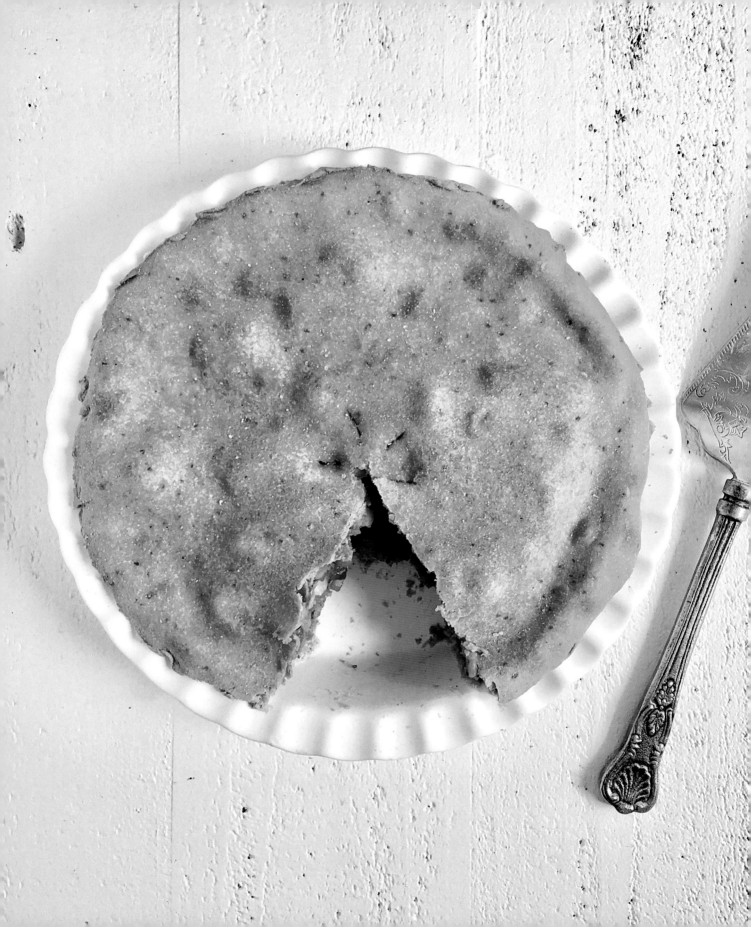

Samosa Pot Pie

MAKES ONE 9-INCH PIE

Everyone loves samosas, and everyone loves pot pie. We decided to marry the two together, and the combination is divine. It is crunchy, filling, and delivers a classic samosa flavor that will explode in your mouth. Our son loves samosas, and he thinks this pie is the bomb!

For the crust

2 cups white whole-wheat pastry flour

1 tsp. ajwain seeds

1 tsp. Himalayan pink salt

1 Tbsp. coconut sugar

½ cup coconut oil

½ cup ice-cold water

1 Preheat the oven to 375 degrees F.

2 Place all the crust ingredients into a food processor and blend until a dough forms. Divide the dough into thirds.

3 Sprinkle flour on a clean, dry surface and roll out ⅔ of the dough into a circle shape about 3 inches larger than a 9-inch pie dish.

4 Carefully transfer the dough circle to a 9-inch pie dish, allowing the edge of the dough to rest over the pie dish rim. Use a fork to punch holes around the inside bottom of the piecrust so that the steam is released when the pie is baking.

5 With the reserved dough, roll out a circle the width of the pie dish. This will be the covering for the pie once it is filled.

Samosa Pot Pie (*cont.*)

For the filling

2 Tbsp. coconut oil

1 tsp. garam masala

1 tsp. mustard seeds

½ tsp. coriander

¼ tsp. ginger powder

¼ tsp. turmeric

1 tsp. ajwain seeds

½ tsp. cumin seeds

1½ tsp. Himalayan pink salt

¼ cup minced red onion

1 tsp. minced garlic

5 cups peeled and cubed potatoes, boiled

½ cup chopped carrots

1 cup peas

1 Heat the coconut oil in a large pan and add in all the spices and salt, followed by the onions and garlic. Stir together and sauté for 2–3 minutes. Then add the potatoes, carrots, and peas and cook for an additional 2–3 minutes.

2 Spoon the filling into the piecrust and cover with the second circle of dough. Fold the edge of the bottom dough circle over the edge of the top circle and form a ridge with your fingers. Poke holes in the top circle with a fork.

3 Bake the Samosa Pot Pie in the oven for 30–40 minutes, or until the top is golden brown.

4 Serve with Cashew Cream Everything Sauce (page 198) and Avocado Mint Chutney (page 195).

Mama's Stuffed Shells

SERVES 4–6

When people think of plant-based cuisine, a common fear is that they will lose some of their favorite foods and that nothing will ever be the same. But you can still enjoy your most beloved meals! This fun, attractive-looking dish is creative, playful, and a joy to make. Our family loves stuffing the shells together, getting messy in the kitchen, and then popping this bad boy into the oven. We are confident this recipe will rival many dairy-rich versions. In fact, most people who try it say these are the best stuffed shells they have ever had. The dish is rich, creamy, and satisfying to the stomach and taste buds. Mama's Stuffed Shells are full of dietary fiber, protein, iron, minerals, and B vitamins. You can use regular large pasta shells or whole-wheat or gluten-free. Get ready to blow your friends and family away with this one!

Simple Cream Cheese (page 188)

2 Tbsp. olive oil

½ cup diced onion

1 Tbsp. minced garlic

1 tsp. oregano

½ tsp. thyme

2 cups minced cremini mushrooms

½ tsp. Himalayan pink salt

1 cup chopped fresh spinach

1 16-oz. box of large whole-wheat or brown-rice pasta shells

¼ cup minced fresh basil

1 24-oz. jar pasta sauce

Vegan cheese (we like Follow Your Heart mozzarella in the block form)

Mama's Stuffed Shells (cont.)

1. Make Simple Cream Cheese. This can be done the day prior or a couple of hours before you make the meal.

2. Preheat the oven to 375 degrees F.

3. Pour the olive oil into a hot frying pan over medium-to-high heat. Stir in the diced onions, minced garlic, oregano, and thyme and sauté until the onions are soft, about 2–3 minutes. Add mushrooms and salt and cook for another 3–5 minutes, or until the mushrooms are soft and golden. Finally, add chopped spinach and cook for another 2 minutes, until the spinach is soft. Remove from heat and let cool for 15–20 minutes.

4. Boil a large pot of water and follow the cooking instructions on the large pasta shells box. Drain and rinse the cooked shells with cool water so they retain a small amount of durability.

5. Add the Simple Cream Cheese and minced fresh basil to the mushroom and spinach mixture and stir to combine. Spoon into a pastry bag or a large Ziploc bag with one corner cut off.

6. Spread a small amount of pasta sauce on the bottom of a lasagna tray. One by one, squeeze the creamy mushroom-spinach mixture into each shell and lay the shell in the tray. Drizzle more pasta sauce over the top. Then grate some vegan cheese on top.

7. Bake in the oven for 30 minutes. Enjoy!

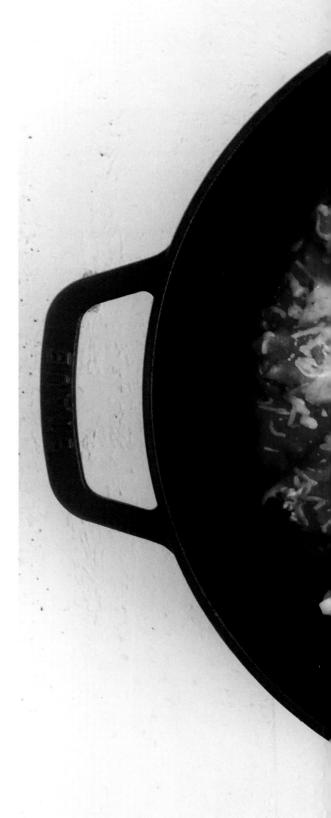

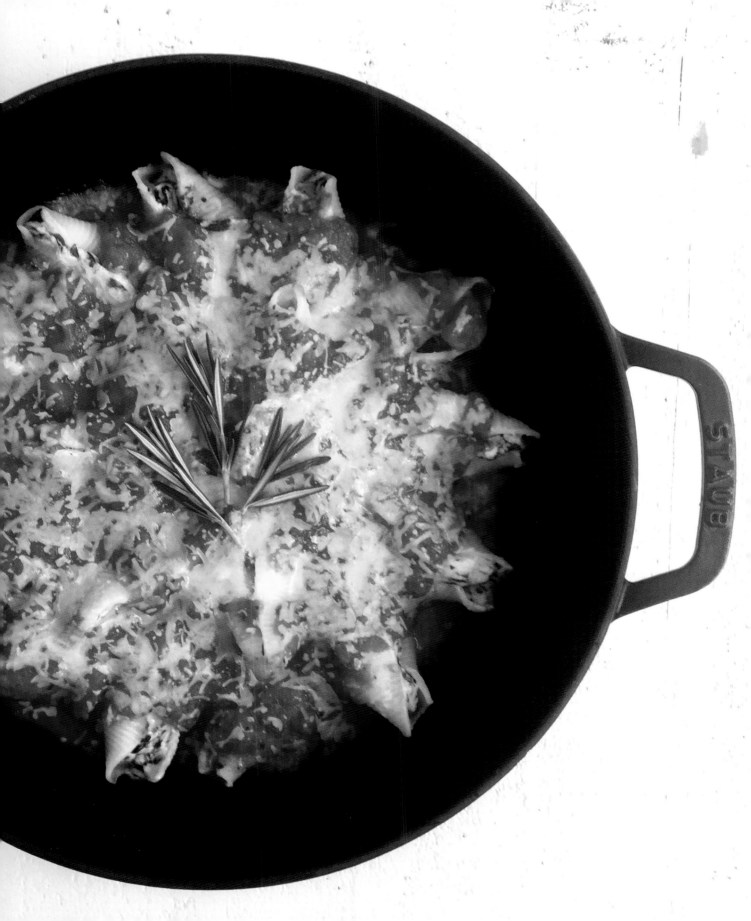

The One and Only Black Bean Burger

MAKES 6–8 PATTIES

Leftovers can lead you to all sorts of surprising culinary delights. We made these delicious black bean burgers one day because we wanted to use up some leftover brown rice. We love how these burgers won't break apart like other veggie burgers. Plus they're filled with wholesome plant food, like sweet potatoes, black beans, kale, and flax meal. Your kids won't even realize how many veggies they're eating! You can also melt vegan cheese on top of them (we like the Follow Your Heart brand, made with coconut oil). You can even serve it on top of a salad. There are endless combinations for this hearty burger.

1 garlic clove, peeled

½ small onion, coarsely chopped

1 can black beans, rinsed and drained

⅓ cup shredded kale

2 Tbsp. chopped cilantro or parsley

⅓ cup shredded raw sweet potato

1 tsp. Himalayan pink salt

1 Tbsp. olive oil

1 Tbsp. tamari

¼ cup oat flour

¼ cup bread crumbs

1 flax egg (page 56)

1½ cups cooked brown rice

Toppings of choice (optional)

1 Preheat the oven to 350 degrees F. Line a large baking sheet with parchment paper.

2 In a small food processor, chop the garlic. Then add the onion and chop again. Next, add the black beans and process until most of them are blended, but leave some chunks for a little texture. Add shredded kale and cilantro or parsley, process the mixture again, and then pour it into a large bowl.

3 Add the shredded sweet potato to the mixture. Stir in the salt, olive oil, tamari, oat flour, and bread crumbs. Next, blend in the flax egg. Lastly, add the brown rice and mix in well.

4 Wet your hands and, with a ⅓- to ½-cup measuring cup (depending on how big you want your burgers), scoop out enough black bean mixture to form into a patty. Flatten on the parchment paper–lined baking sheet so it looks like a burger. Repeat until the mixture is used up.

5 Bake in the oven for 15 minutes, flip the burgers, and bake for another 15 minutes. Remove from the oven and let cool for 5–10 minutes.

6 Top with avocado, tomato, vegan mayonnaise, ketchup, onions, mustard, or whatever your heart desires.

7 These burgers will store well in the fridge for 3–4 days. To reheat, melt a small amount of coconut oil in a frying pan and cook on the stovetop for 3 minutes on each side.

Since there is sweet potato in the burger, we like to chop up the unused potato and bake the pieces at the same time we bake the burgers, then add them on top of the burgers or eat them on the side.

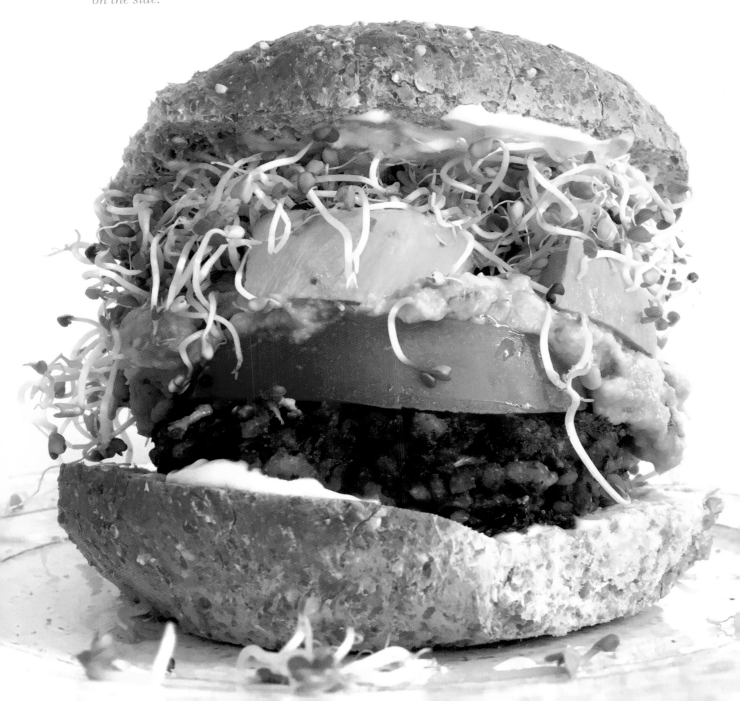

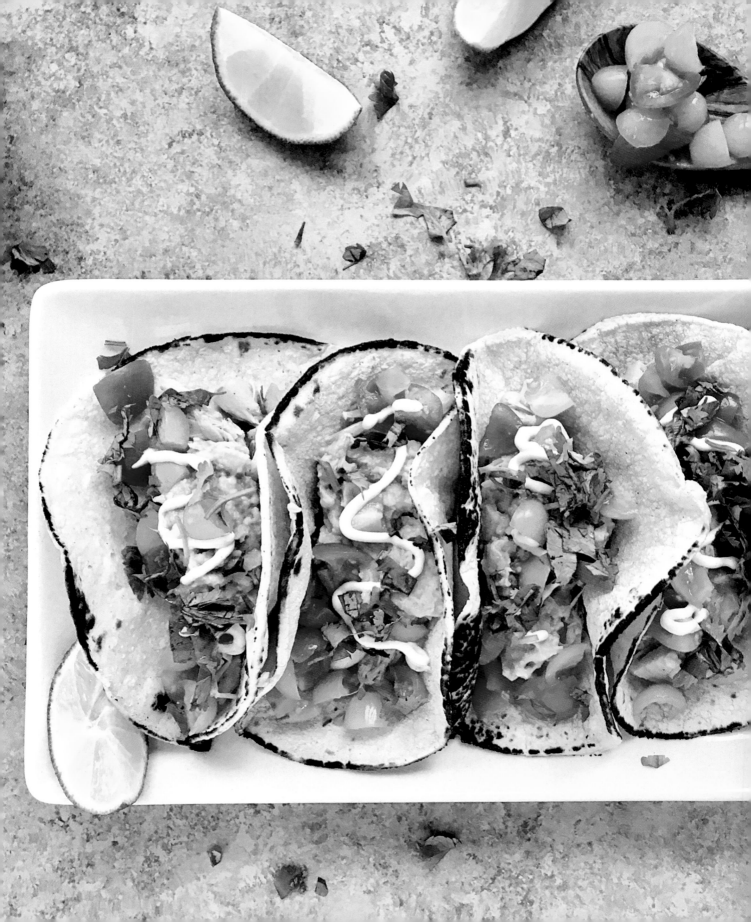

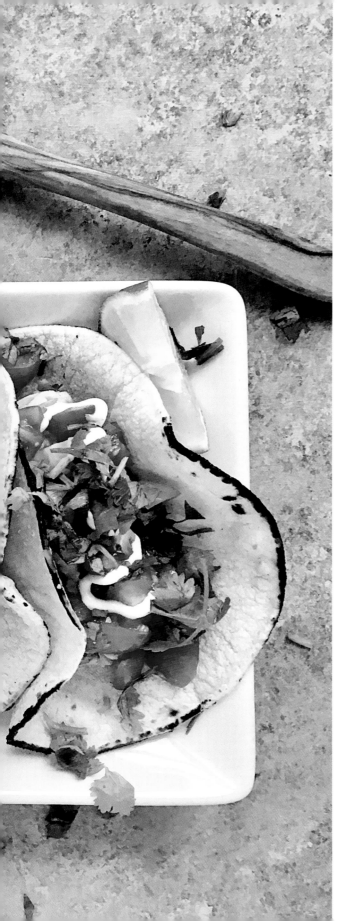

We Love Jackfruit Tacos

SERVES 4

To love someone is to feed them delicious, wholesome food. When these tacos are on the dinner table, you'll feel the love. They are nourishing and satisfying. Our We Love Jackfruit Tacos are loaded with nutrients and full of flavor. They deliver dietary fiber, vitamin B, vitamin A, and protein. Our son loves Mexican food, and this is one of his all-time favorite meals.

For the filling

1 20-oz. can jackfruit

1 Tbsp. coconut oil

½ cup onion

1 tsp. garlic

1 tsp. cumin

½ tsp. oregano

½ tsp. paprika

¼ tsp. chili powder, or to taste

½ tsp. Himalayan pink salt

2 Tbsp. almond butter

½ cup chopped tomato

1 Tbsp. maple syrup

½ Tbsp. soy sauce

1 tsp. vinegar

▶

We Love Jackfruit Tacos *(cont.)*

For the tacos

8 corn tortillas

Guacamole

Salsa

Shredded lettuce

Cashew Cream Everything Sauce (page 198)

Fresh lime wedges

1 Open the jackfruit can and drain the water out, then pour the fruit into a bowl and break up with your hands — it should pull apart easily. Set it aside.

2 Heat the coconut oil in a skillet and toss in the onions, garlic, cumin, oregano, paprika, and chili powder. Sauté for 2–3 minutes, or until the onions are tender.

3 Add the jackfruit and salt and cook, stirring, for 5–8 minutes, or until mixture is tender and well combined.

4 Stir in the almond butter, chopped tomato, maple syrup, soy sauce, and vinegar and cook for another 1–2 minutes.

5 Turn off the heat. To serve, spoon a little filling into a corn tortilla with guacamole, salsa, shredded lettuce, and Cashew Cream Everything Sauce and squeeze fresh lime juice over everything.

Poblano Mexicano Tofu

SERVES 4

There are lots of jokes about how bland tofu is, but tofu's superpower is that it can take on any flavor — it soaks in whatever you put on it. All of the flavors, particularly from the poblano peppers, really shine in this dish. It's spicy but balanced. It'll be the superdish at your next dinner party!

4 raw poblano peppers

1 16-oz. package organic extra-firm tofu

2 Tbsp. grape-seed oil or coconut oil

½ cup minced onion

1 garlic clove, peeled and minced

½ tsp. cumin

¾ tsp. Himalayan pink salt

½ cup Cashew Cream Everything Sauce (page 198)

Juice of ½ lime

Tortillas or rice (optional)

Toppings of choice (optional)

1 Preheat the oven to 550 degrees F.

2 Place poblano peppers on a baking sheet and roast for 15 minutes.

3 While the peppers are roasting, slice the tofu into 1-inch pieces. Heat a large skillet on medium high, add 1 Tbsp. of the grape-seed or coconut oil and the tofu slices, and sauté for 2–3 minutes, then flip to brown the other side. Once the tofu slices are golden brown, place in a bowl and set aside.

4 Keeping the skillet hot, add the remaining 1 Tbsp. grape-seed or coconut oil, onions, garlic, and cumin. Sauté for 2–3 minutes, or until the onions are tender.

5 As soon as the peppers are done roasting, remove from the oven, set them in a bowl, and cover with a lid for 1–2 minutes. This will allow the skins to separate from the peppers. Peel the skins off, remove the seeds, and chop the peppers into 1-inch slices. If you want a spicier dish, keep the seeds in.

6 Add the chopped peppers, tofu slices, and salt to the skillet with the sautéed onions. Over medium heat, stir together until combined.

7 Turn the burner off and add the Cashew Cream Everything Sauce and lime juice. Mix well.

8 Serve in a tortilla with guacamole, salsa, more Cashew Cream Everything Sauce (page 198), and shredded lettuce. Or serve over a bed of brown rice with guacamole, salsa, Cashew Cream Everything Sauce, and diced lettuce to make a Mexican bowl.

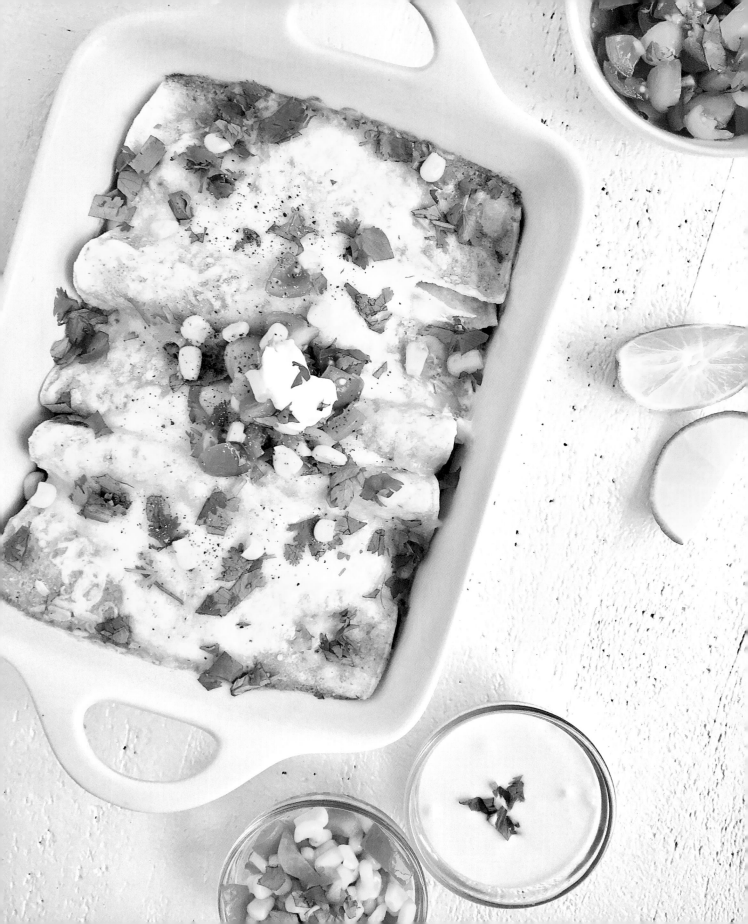

Green Machine Enchiladas

MAKES ONE 9x12 TRAY

When it comes to making enchiladas, it is really all about the sauce. The sauce defines the flavor, so it's not surprising that it's the most complicated part of the meal. The assembly and other aspects of vegan cheese and garnishes are relatively simple to accomplish. Not everyone in our family likes red sauce, so we came up with a green alternative that is incredibly refreshing and light.

For the sauce

2 cups chopped fresh tomatillos

½ cup chopped poblano pepper

2 cups water

½ cup diced red onion

1 tsp. minced garlic

1 tsp. Himalayan pink salt

1 tsp. oregano

1 tsp. cumin

½ cup chopped cilantro

¼ cup pumpkin seeds

1   Place the tomatillos, poblano peppers, and water in a pot and boil for 5 minutes, or until the tomatillos are soft.

2   Pour the contents of the pot into a high-powered blender. Add the onion, garlic, salt, oregano, cumin, cilantro, and pumpkin seeds and blend for 30–45 seconds, or until smooth.

3   Pour around ¼ cup of the green enchilada sauce on the bottom of a casserole pan and spread it around so it reaches each end of the pan.

▶

Green Machine Enchiladas (*cont.*)

For the enchiladas

2 Tbsp. coconut oil, plus oil for toasting tortillas

12–15 corn tortillas

2 cups chopped red, orange, or yellow bell peppers

½ tsp. minced garlic

¼ tsp. Himalayan pink salt

2 cups corn

2 cups cooked black beans

Vegan cheese (we like Follow Your Heart mozzarella in the block form)

1 Preheat the oven to 425 degrees F.

2 Heat a skillet over medium-high heat. Add ¼ tsp. coconut oil, slide on a tortilla, and toast for a few seconds on each side, or until it is soft. Set aside and repeat until you have enough tortillas to fill the casserole pan with enchiladas.

3 Add 1 Tbsp. coconut oil to the skillet, then add the chopped bell peppers, garlic, and half of the salt. Sauté over medium-high heat for 2–3 minutes, or until tender. Set the cooked bell peppers aside.

4 Keeping the skillet hot, add in another 1 Tbsp. of coconut oil, the corn, and the remaining salt. Cook for 2–3 minutes, or until the corn is soft. Turn off the heat.

5 Scoop about 2 Tbsp. beans into a tortilla, followed by bell peppers, corn, and a slice of vegan cheese. Roll the tortilla up and set in the casserole dish. Repeat until the entire pan is filled.

6 Pour the remaining green enchilada sauce over the tortillas. You can also drizzle some Cashew Cream Everything Sauce (page 198) and sprinkle shredded vegan cheese over the top.

7 Bake in the oven for 15–20 minutes. Serve hot.

Asian Cowboy BBQ Tofu

SERVES 4

The reason we call this dish the Asian Cowboy BBQ Tofu is because we're using tofu for Southern-style cooking. It's a fusion of great, smoky BBQ flavor with an Eastern protein. This unique home-style BBQ dish is Tamal's own creation. It has the tangy, spicy, salty, sweet, finger-licking goodness Southern BBQ should have—just without the refined sugars, dyes, and preservatives! We love making Southern-inspired bowls, filled with our Asian Cowboy BBQ Tofu, mashed potatoes, and green beans.

For the BBQ sauce

½ cup organic ketchup

1 tsp. apple cider vinegar

1 tsp. vegan Worcestershire sauce

1 Tbsp. maple syrup

½ tsp. yellow mustard

½ tsp. blackstrap molasses

½ tsp. paprika

½ tsp. garlic powder

½ tsp. onion powder

1 Tbsp. peanut butter (optional)

For the tofu

2 tsp. coconut oil

1 15.5-oz. package firm tofu, cubed

1 In a medium-size bowl, combine all the ingredients for the BBQ sauce except the peanut butter and mix well.

2 Add peanut butter, if using, and stir well with a whisk, so it becomes part of the mixture. The peanut butter is not essential to the BBQ sauce, but it gives the tofu a really nice, creamy flavor. This should make about ¾ cup of BBQ sauce.

3 Heat a cast-iron or nonstick skillet over medium heat, add the coconut oil and cubed tofu, and sauté until the cubes are golden brown. Then flip them to cook on the other side.

4 Turn the burner off, add the BBQ sauce to the cooked tofu, and toss until the cubes are very well coated. Serve with Cauliflower Mash (page 98) and greens.

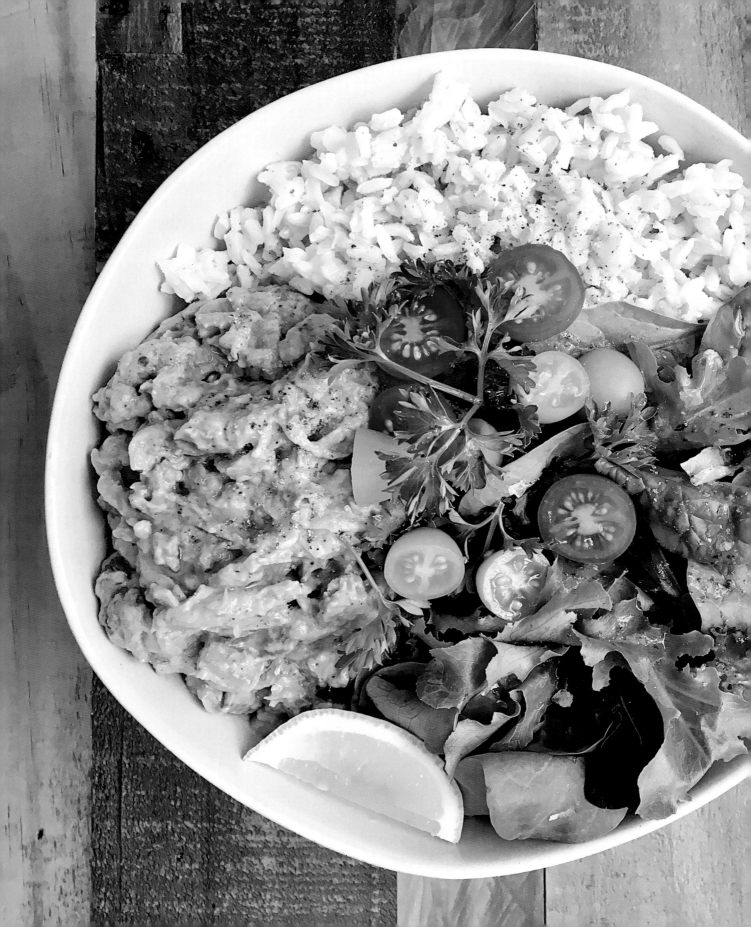

Eggplant Curry

SERVES 4–6

If you like Indian food, our Eggplant Curry will have you coming back for seconds. There are so many layers of flavors to enjoy! This curry is amazing on a bed of warm brown rice or in a wrap with baby greens. We love to eat it on cold nights when we want something filling and comforting. This curry works well for lunch, too. It's healthy and energizing, so it won't leave you with an early-afternoon food coma.

4 eggplants

1 tsp. Himalayan pink salt plus a few pinches

2 tsp. olive oil

2 Tbsp. coconut oil

½ cup chopped red onion

1 tsp. minced garlic

1 tsp. curry powder

2 tsp. cumin

⅛ tsp. ginger powder

⅛ tsp. paprika

¼ tsp. turmeric powder

½ tsp. garam masala

¼ cup diced sun-dried tomatoes

¼ cup almond butter

½ cup Cashew Cream Everything Sauce (page 198)

1 Preheat the oven to 400 degrees F. Line a baking sheet with parchment paper.

2 Cut the eggplants in half lengthwise, then make deep crisscross patterns on the inside of each eggplant half with a knife. Sprinkle a pinch of salt over the patterns, making sure to get it into the creases. The salt will help pull the moisture out of the eggplant and expedite the cooking process. Place the eggplant halves face down on the baking sheet and let them sit for 30 minutes. Then drizzle about ½ tsp. of olive oil over the crisscross pattern of each half and spread the oil around the open face.

3 Turn the eggplants face down again on the baking sheet and roast in the oven for 30–40 minutes, or until they are soft and have the classic roasted look. Let them cool.

4 With a spoon, scrape the inside of each eggplant into a bowl. You should have roughly 5 cups of roasted eggplant. Set aside.

5 Place coconut oil in a medium pot and add onions, garlic, and the spices (holding off on the remaining salt). Sauté, stirring, for 3–5 minutes, or until the onions are soft. Add sun-dried tomatoes and cook for another 3–5 minutes.

6 Stir in the roasted eggplant, almond butter, Cashew Cream Everything Sauce, and remaining 1 tsp. salt. Cook for another 2–3 minutes, then serve.

Hella Falafels

MAKES ABOUT 12 FALAFELS

Falafels are delicious, but traditionally they are deep-fried and bean heavy and are best enjoyed on special occasions. Our family loves to eat them often, so we came up with this lighter variation. We use zucchini in lieu of beans and just a bit of oil to fry them. These falafels are high in protein and packed with nutrients. You can make Hella Falafels regularly, without any guilt. They disappear quickly whenever we have a Mediterranean night at our house. They're so satisfying and flavorful!

1 cup garbanzo bean flour

1 tsp. cumin

1 tsp. Himalayan pink salt

1 tsp. oregano

½ tsp. baking soda

2 medium zucchini

½ cup shredded fresh basil

1 tsp. minced garlic

½ cup olive oil

2 Tbsp. grape-seed
or coconut oil

Toppings of choice (optional)

1   In a medium-size bowl, place the garbanzo bean flour, cumin, salt, oregano, and baking soda and stir together until they are combined.

2   Grate the zucchini into a bowl. Squeeze out the excess water with your hands. Add 2 cups of the grated zucchini to the dry mixture and mix together thoroughly.

3   Mix in shredded fresh basil, minced garlic, and olive oil, combining until a dough forms. On a clean, dry work surface, roll dough into 1-inch balls and then flatten them like pancakes with a spatula.

4   Heat a large nonstick pan on high and add 2 Tbsp. grape-seed or coconut oil. Place the falafel pancakes in the hot oil and fry for 1 minute on each side, or until golden brown. We like to press the falafels down with a spatula once we have flipped them. This way the zucchini gets cooked really well.

5   Serve with a salad or in a pita, with toppings like Magic Tahini Sauce (page 189), chopped tomatoes, kalamata olives, and chopped cucumbers.

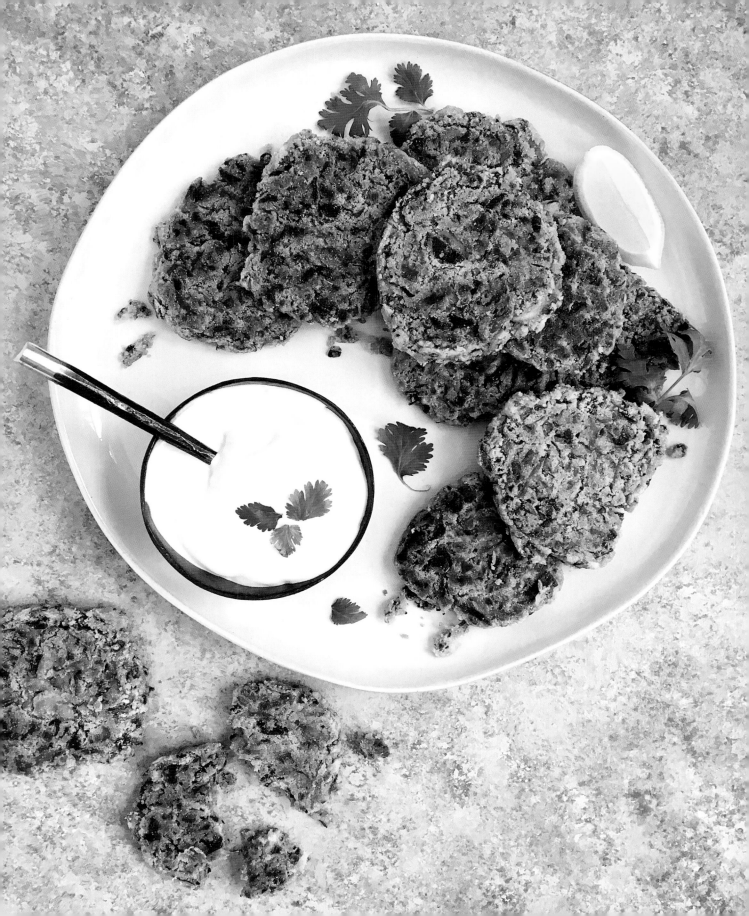

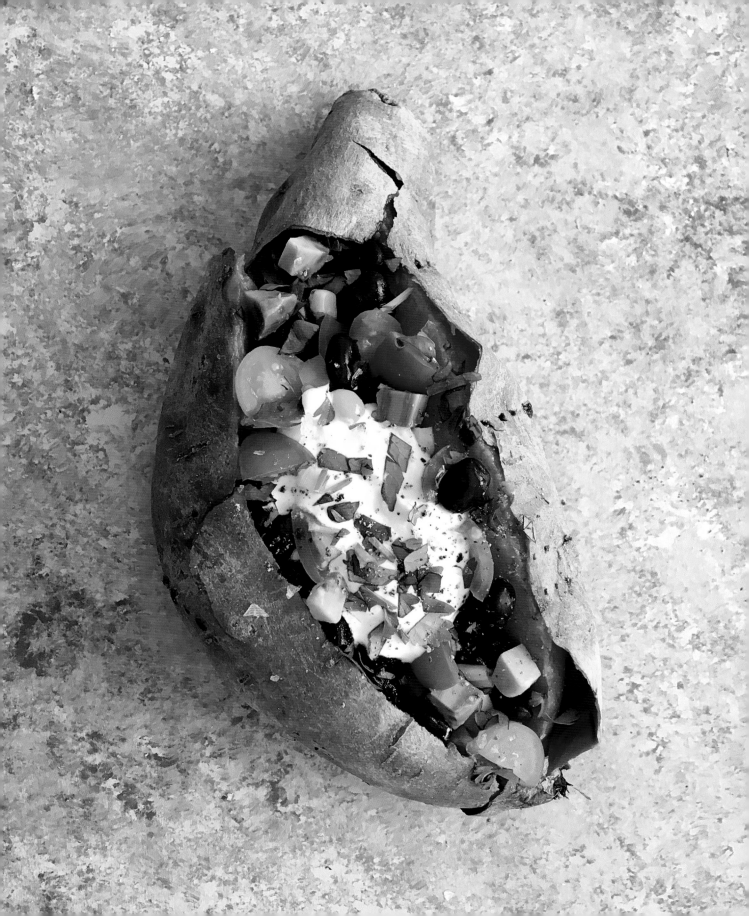

Stuffed Mexican Sweet Potato

SERVES 4

When we're thinking about what to put on the menu for an upcoming dinner party, this delicious dish often comes up. It even looks festive, with all of its colorful ingredients. This gluten-free Mexican dinner is filling but not heavy. It is loaded with fiber, potassium, protein, and good fats. The flavors strike a perfect balance, too. Sweet potato offsets black beans and the zest of our lime corn. Together they create a mouthwatering combination of full-bodied flavor and plate appeal.

4 large sweet potatoes

1 Tbsp. coconut oil

¼ cup diced red onion

1 cup corn (fresh or frozen)

½ Tbsp. lime juice

⅛ tsp. pepper

¼ tsp. Himalayan pink salt

Coconut oil and pinch of salt (for garnishing the potatoes)

1 cup cooked salted black beans (canned or homemade)

Salsa

Guacamole

Cashew Cream Everything Sauce (page 198)

1   Preheat the oven to 400 degrees F. Line a medium-size baking sheet with parchment paper.

2   Wash the sweet potatoes and puncture holes in their skins with a fork. Place the potatoes on the parchment paper-lined baking sheet and bake in the oven for 45–55 minutes, or until they are cooked all the way through.

3   While the sweet potatoes are baking, heat 1 Tbsp. coconut oil in a small pot and throw in your red onions. Sauté for 1–2 minutes, or until they are tender. Add the frozen or fresh corn and cook for an additional 3–5 minutes, or until the corn is tender. Mix in the lime juice, black pepper, and salt and turn off the heat.

4   When the sweet potatoes are done, remove from the oven and slice each one down the middle with a knife to create a classic baked-potato opening. Lightly garnish each potato with coconut oil and salt. Then top with the lime corn mixture, black beans, salsa, guacamole, and Cashew Cream Everything Sauce. Serve right away, while the potatoes are still warm.

The trick to making this recipe fast and easy is having Cashew Cream Everything Sauce already stocked in the refrigerator and cooked beans on hand.

Masala Dosa

SERVES 4–6

Indian food was a staple for Tamal growing up in a yoga ashram. His parents loved cooking Vedic food and taught all of their children the culinary arts of India. Tamal loves masala dosa, but traditionally it requires using white rice and vegetable oil. He modified this recipe with whole-grain brown rice, urad dal (black lentils that are husked and split, so they are yellow in color for this recipe), and extra-virgin coconut oil to create a variation so light and crispy, you can't tell it's been modified at all. The only difference is how you feel after you eat it. Rather than becoming tired enough to take a nap, you'll feel like working out or getting things accomplished. This dish delivers a perfect protein with good fats. In short, Tamal's recipe is scrumptious *and* energizing! The batter needs to be prepared one day before you will be serving the dish.

1 cup long-grain brown rice (preferably jasmine)

½ cup urad dal

4 cups water

½ tsp. fenugreek

1 tsp. Himalayan pink salt

Coconut oil for cooking

Samosa Pot Pie filling (page 154)

1   Rinse the rice and dal. Soak in a bowl with 4 cups of water for 8–10 hours.

2   Drain the rice-dal mixture over a bowl, reserving the water it soaked in. Place the mixture in a food processor with 1½ cups of the soaking water and the fenugreek and salt. Blend until smooth. It should look like pancake batter.

3   Pour the dosa batter into a bowl, cover, and let it sit at room temperature in a dark place for 10–15 hours to ferment.

4   Pour ¼ cup of the batter into a large nonstick pan and spread into a thin circle with the back of a spoon. After cooking over medium-high heat for about 1 minute, you will see the dough is not wet anymore on the top side. Lightly brush ¼ tsp. of coconut oil on the top side and cook for 1 more minute, or until you see the dosa browning through the bottom and it looks crispy — that's how you'll know it's ready. (Only cook on one side.) Remove from the pan with a large spatula and set on a serving plate. We like to make one dosa at a time and serve it hot immediately.

5   To serve, fill the dosa with the filling from the Samosa Pot Pie recipe (page 154), fold it in half, and top it with Cashew Cream Everything Sauce (page 198) and Avocado Mint Chutney (page 195). Repeat the dosa-making process until all the batter is used.

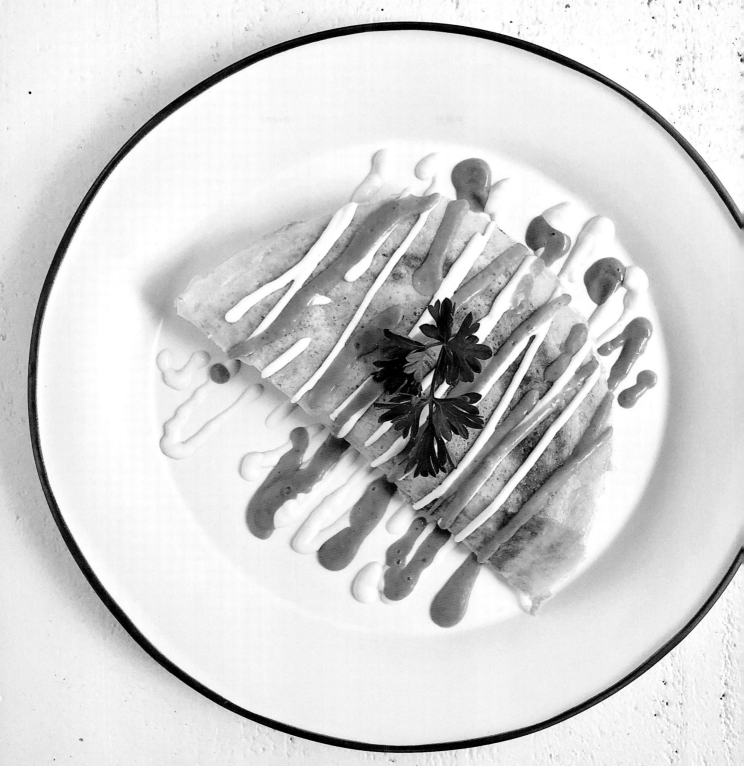

*This dish requires 8–10 hours of
soaking and sprouting time for the rice and dal.
Be sure to allow for this time when preparing it.*

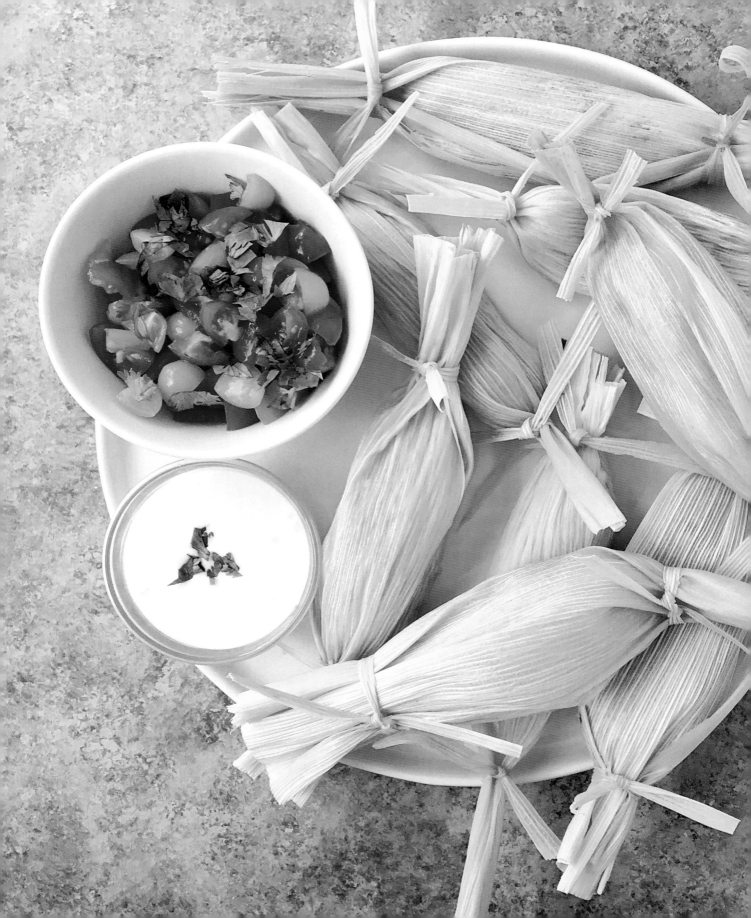

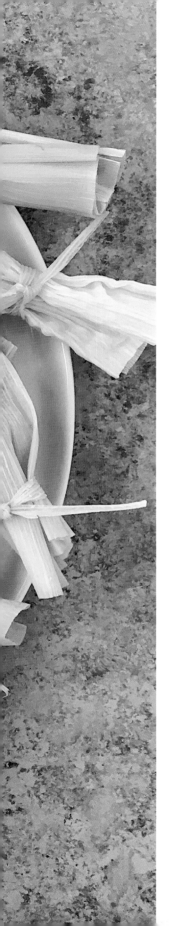

Tamal's Sweet Potato and Apple Tamales

MAKES ABOUT 10 TAMALES

Throughout Tamal's life, people used to jokingly call him Hot Tamale, just to have a little fun with him. The irony is that Tamal makes really good hot tamales of all sorts, with ingredients you might not even expect. This sweet potato, apple, and cheese tamale will delight your palate. We love the flavor combination, but you can use just about any filling you like with this recipe: cheese and corn, sautéed tofu and cheese . . . the list goes on and on. We like to use Follow Your Heart vegan cheese and to pour our Cashew Cream Everything Sauce (page 198) and our Oaxaca Mole Sauce (page 191) over these tamales to give them a spicy, creamy boost.

10 tamale corn husks

1 large sweet potato

1 apple

⅓ cup vegan mozzarella cheese, cut into strips 2 inches long and ¼ inch wide

3 cups masa flour, such as Bob's Red Mill

1 tsp. baking powder

1 tsp. Himalayan pink salt

5 Tbsp. melted extra-virgin coconut oil

2 cups water

1 Place the corn husks in a large bowl of hot water. Let them soak for 30 minutes, until they become soft.

2 While the husks are soaking, peel the sweet potato and cut into slices 2 inches long and ½ inch wide. Cook the sweet potato slices in boiling water for 8–10 minutes, or until tender. Drain, add a pinch of salt, and set aside.

3 Peel and core the apple. Cut into slices identical to the sweet potato slices and set aside. Do the same with the vegan cheese.

4 Place masa flour, baking powder, and salt in a food processor and blitz for 10 seconds, until combined. Pour in the melted coconut oil and water and blitz again for 20–30 seconds, or until the mixture forms a dough.

▶

Tamal's Sweet Potato and Apple Tamales *(cont.)*

To assemble the tamales

1 On a clean cutting board, pat dry a single corn husk with a towel. Open the corn husk with the narrow end pointing toward you and the wider end pointing away from you. Spread a 2-inch ball of masa dough with a spoon along the inside of the corn husk, leaving 1–2 inches of the narrow end of the corn husk empty.

2 Lay 1 slice of sweet potato, 2 slices of apple, and 1 slice of cheese over the masa dough. Don't overfill.

3 Fold the left and right sides of the corn husk inward so the masa dough connects and fully encases the sweet potato, apple, and cheese slices. Next, pinch and twist the narrow end, then fold the narrow end up toward the wide end. Place in a steamer basket. Repeat until all the dough and filling are used up.

4 Place the steamer basket with the tamales in a large pot filled with 3 inches of water. Bring to a boil, cover the tamales with a lid, turn the burner down to a medium heat, and steam for 30 minutes.

Soul Bowl

SERVES 4

If you love smoky black-eyed peas, sweet corn bread, and garlic-flavored collard greens, then our Soul Bowl is for you! Inspired by soulful Southern cooking, it's packed with nutrients as well as texture, color, and comfort. When it is cold and rainy outside, we whip up our Soul Bowl. We've worked hard to refine this dish and to strike the perfect balance of sweet flavors and hearty textures in the corn bread. The final version has a perfectly authentic, rustic feel. The black-eyed peas are salty and savory, and they offset the sweetness of the corn bread. The collards are the ultimate Southern green to pair with this playful bowl.

For the black-eyed peas

2 Tbsp. grape-seed oil

2 Tbsp. garbanzo bean flour

½ cup chopped onion

1 tsp. minced garlic

½ cup diced tomato

½ cup diced carrot

½ cup diced bell pepper

½ cup shredded zucchini

1½ cups canned black-eyed peas, drained and rinsed

3 bay leaves

½ tsp. pepper

¼ tsp. red chili flakes

1 tsp. cumin

1 tsp. Himalayan pink salt

2 Tbsp. nutritional yeast

2 cups vegetable broth

1 Tbsp. apple cider vinegar

½ tsp. liquid smoke

1 In a medium-size pot over medium heat, add the oil and garbanzo bean flour and cook, stirring constantly, for 1 minute.

2 Add onion and garlic, then sauté for 1–2 minutes.

3 Add tomato, carrot, bell pepper, zucchini, and black-eyed peas. Sauté for 2–3 minutes.

4 Stir in the bay leaves, pepper, red chili flakes, cumin, salt, and nutritional yeast. Add the vegetable broth, apple cider vinegar, and liquid smoke, and stir again. Bring mixture to a boil, then turn the flame down. Cook at a rolling simmer for 5–10 minutes, or until the vegetables are tender.

▶

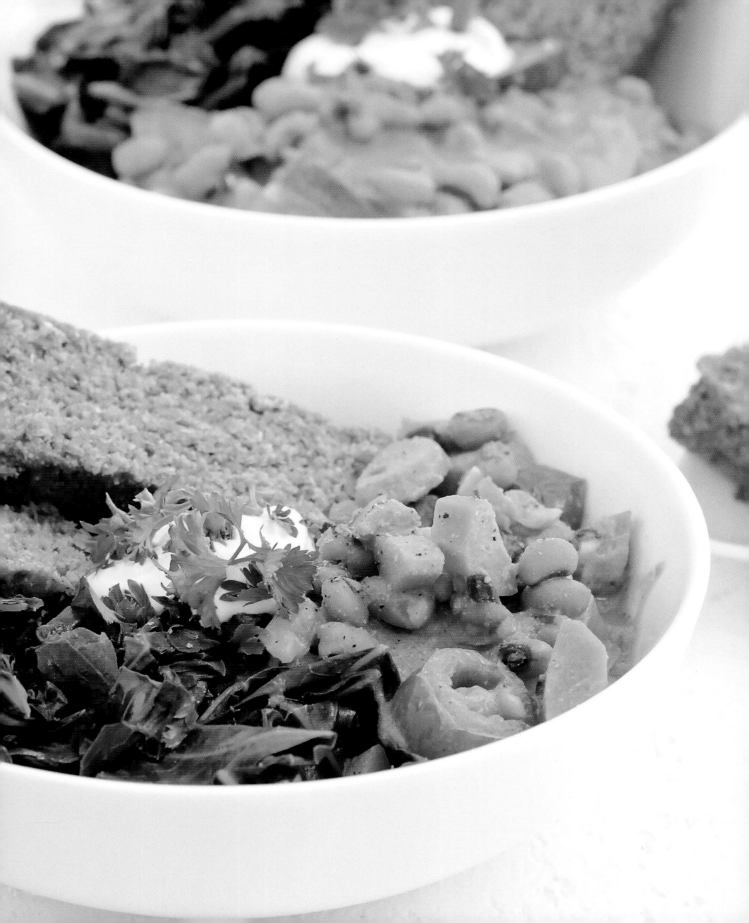

Soul Bowl (*cont.*)

For the corn bread

1 cup cornmeal

1 cup white whole-wheat pastry flour

1 Tbsp. baking powder

½ tsp. Himalayan pink salt

½ cup coconut sugar

½ cup melted coconut oil

1 flax egg (page 56)

¾ cup unsweetened nondairy milk

1 Tbsp. apple cider vinegar

. . . .

1 Preheat the oven to 400 degrees F. Grease the inside of a loaf pan with coconut oil.

2 Mix cornmeal, white whole-wheat pastry flour, baking powder, salt, and coconut sugar in a medium-size bowl until well combined.

3 Add coconut oil, flax egg, nondairy milk, and apple cider vinegar to the dry ingredients and combine until a batter forms.

4 Pour the batter into the prepared loaf pan. Bake in the oven for 25 minutes, or until the top of the corn bread is light golden brown.

For the collard greens

1 tsp. grape-seed oil

1 tsp. minced garlic

8 cups chopped collard greens

1 tsp. Himalayan pink salt

¼ cup water

. . . .

1 Heat the grape-seed oil in a large pot or cast-iron skillet. Add garlic and sauté for 1 minute over medium heat.

2 Add collard greens and salt. Continue to cook, stirring continuously, for 3–5 minutes, or until the collard greens reduce in size and start to become soft.

3 Add the water, cover the pot or skillet, and simmer for 5–8 minutes.

4 To serve, place a slice of corn bread in a bowl with a scoop of the black-eyed peas, and then add the collard greens on the side.

Fakin' Bacon BLT

SERVES 4

If you love the smoky, salty, sweet flavor of bacon, then this tempeh variation is for you. Fakin' Bacon can be used not only in BLTs but also on Hawaiian pizza or as a side with scrambled tofu. It's a simple dish, but the preparation requires a little bit of patience. The slow, overnight marinating process is worth it, because that's where all the flavor comes in. We like to make double batches so we have leftovers (if we can manage not to eat it all at once!).

1 7.5-oz package tempeh, cut into ¼-inch strips

2 Tbsp. soy sauce

2 Tbsp. maple syrup

1 Tbsp. balsamic vinegar

1 Tbsp. olive oil

½ tsp. liquid smoke

¼ tsp. paprika

½ tsp. garlic powder

½ tsp. onion powder

Oil for frying

1 Boil 1 cup of water in a pot or skillet. Add the tempeh strips, cover the pot or skillet with a lid, and turn the heat down to a simmer for 5 minutes. Remove the tempeh pieces from the water and lay them on a dry towel to air out.

2 As the tempeh dries, make the marinade by whisking together the remaining ingredients in a medium-size bowl until combined.

3 Set the tempeh pieces in a medium-size Tupperware container, then pour the marinade over them. Cover the container and refrigerate overnight. We like to give a light toss to the tempeh every time we open the refrigerator, to distribute the marinade more actively.

4 The next day, heat a skillet with some oil and fry the tempeh slices over medium heat for 2–3 minutes on each side, or until golden brown.

For a delicious BLT sandwich, serve the tempeh on toasted bread with sliced tomato, avocado, lettuce, and a bit of vegan mayonnaise.

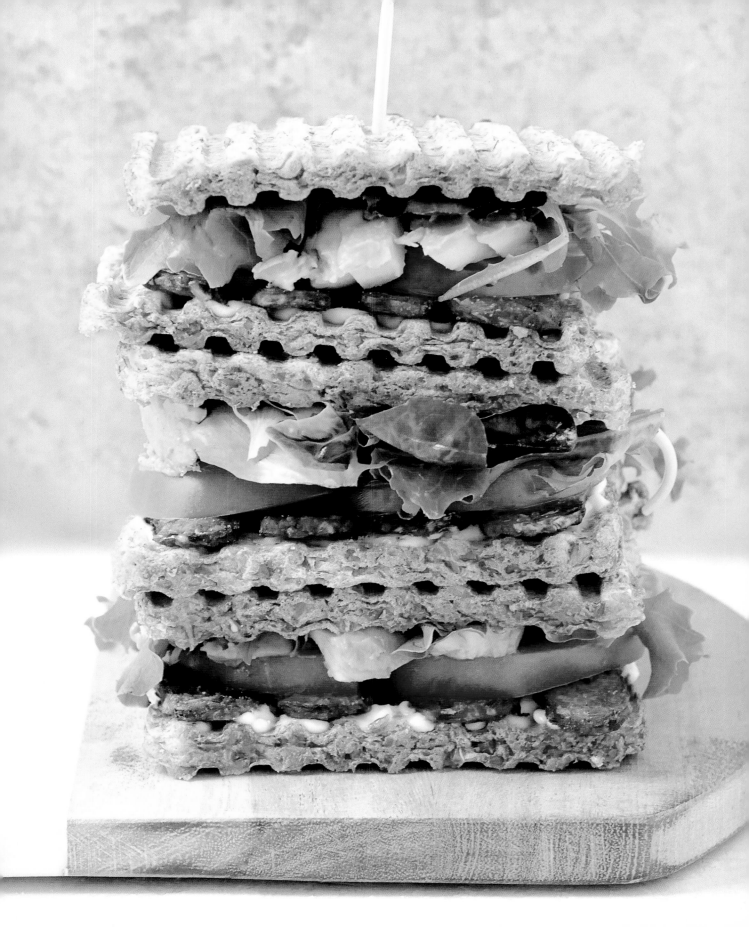

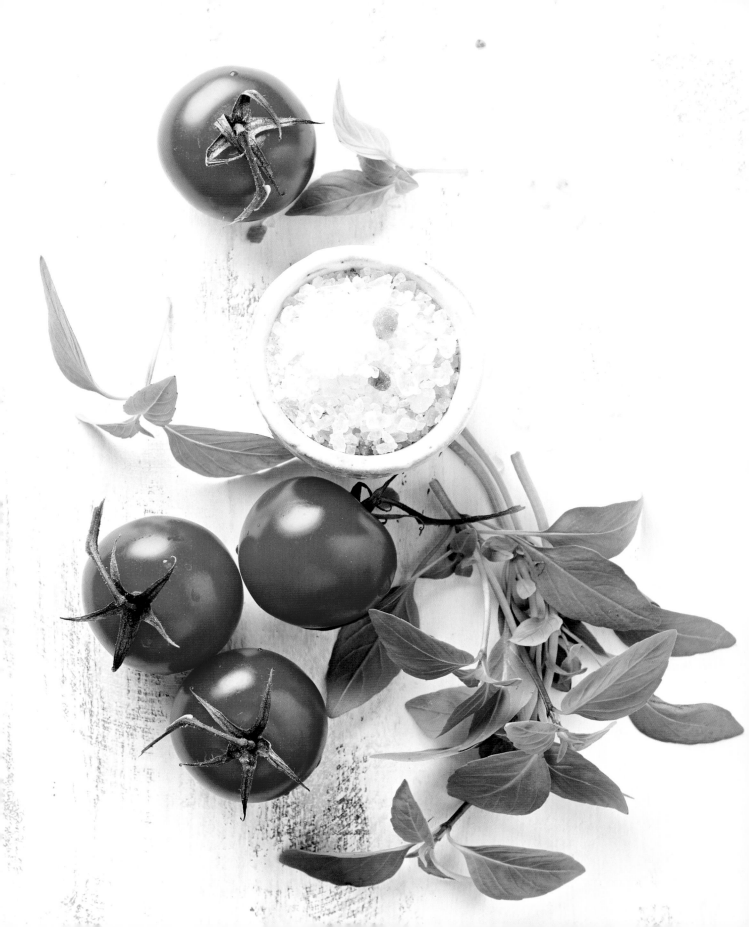

dips and sauces

Vegan Sour Cream

MAKES ABOUT 1½ CUPS

This is *the* best dairy-free sour cream you will ever have! You'll find yourself putting it into regular rotation in your kitchen. Many of the ingredients are probably already in your fridge. It's a dynamic and delicious topping on anything from baked potatoes to tacos. Mix it with a little salsa to make a tasty dip for chips or French fries. You'll never miss the dairy in sour cream again.

1 cup raw cashews, soaked 6–8 hours

¼ cup water

3 Tbsp. lemon juice

1 Tbsp. apple cider vinegar

½ tsp. garlic powder

½ tsp. onion powder

¼ tsp. Himalayan pink salt

1 Place all of the ingredients in a high-speed blender and blend until smooth.

2 Store in the refrigerator for at least 1 hour before serving. This will help thicken it up and give it the best consistency.

Avocado Cilantro Lime Dressing

MAKES 1 CUP

This creamy five-minute dressing will be your new best friend. You will want to pour it on everything for that extra dash of flavor. If you like a little kick, add the jalapeño. If you want to keep it mellow, omit it. The avocado is super creamy and loaded with healthy fats and fiber. The cilantro is an amazing blood detoxifier and purifier. If you have extra Cashew Cream Everything Sauce, use that instead of vegan mayonnaise. This dressing will liven up a Mexican Chop Salad (page 131)—or any salad, for that matter. It's so versatile that if you make it a little on the thicker side, you can even use it as a spread on a veggie wrap, a sandwich, or tacos.

1 avocado, peeled, pitted and roughly chopped

1 cup cilantro

2 Tbsp. fresh lime juice

1 1-inch-long jalapeño pepper (optional)

¼ cup vegan mayonnaise, such as Vegenaise, or Cashew Cream Everything Sauce (page 198)

¼ tsp. Himalayan pink salt

Pepper to taste

¼–½ cup water

1 Blend all ingredients together in a small food processor or blender, starting with ¼ cup water. Add more water gradually until you get your desired consistency.

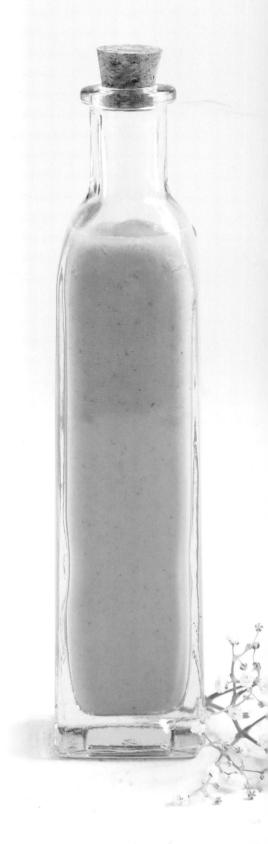

Simple Cream Cheese

MAKES 2 CUPS

Whenever Victoria took Savannah to New York, they'd eat warm fresh bagels with whipped cream cheese, topped off by a cup of hot chocolate. It became a mother-daughter tradition, but they knew it wasn't healthy. So when they adopted a fully plant-based lifestyle, they ditched the white-flour bagels and the dairy cream cheese for good. Our Simple Cream Cheese tastes just like the New York whipped cream cheese, only this nondairy version is incredibly healthy. It is cultured, which means it is loaded with probiotics, as well as good fats and protein. Try it the way we do, on a bagel. You can also spread this on toast, use it to fill your favorite lasagna, or make icing with it for an amazing frosted cake. This cheese can go head-to-head with any dairy product, any day!

1 cup unsweetened nondairy milk

1 cup cashews, soaked for at least 1 hour

1 tsp. garlic powder

¾ tsp. Himalayan pink salt

1 Tbsp. fresh lemon juice

½ cup water

½ tsp. agar powder

1 Blend all of the ingredients except the water and the agar powder in a high-powered blender for 45 seconds, or until smooth.

2 In a small pot, boil ½ cup water with ½ tsp. agar powder, then turn off heat and let the mixture thicken for about 5 minutes.

3 Add the water and agar powder mixture to the smooth cashew cream in the blender and blend for another 30 seconds.

4 Pour into small cheesecake pans and refrigerate for at least 30 minutes before serving.

If you don't have small cheesecake pans, any container will work to chill the cream cheese.

Magic Tahini Sauce

MAKES ABOUT 1½ CUPS

This creamy tahini sauce is one of the staples in our house. It's very versatile. We use it on just about anything, from fresh salads and Mediteranean dishes to rice bowls and more. There is no need to feel guilty when devouring this rich, nutrient-dense sauce. It's loaded with lots of B vitamins, vitamins E and K, and minerals like calcium, phosphorus, magnesium, and potassium.

½ cup tahini

½ cup water

¼ cup lemon juice

2 Tbsp. extra-virgin olive oil

¾ tsp. Himalayan pink salt

¼ tsp. minced garlic

1 Tbsp. minced fresh basil

1   Place all ingredients in a high-powered blender and blitz for 45–60 seconds.

Thai Peanut Sauce

Peanut sauce is a must in our house, because we love making summer rolls and Asian salads. If you dropped by our house on a Sunday, you'd probably find us making this sauce. We take that time to prepare it ahead so that we can have it on hand all week long. And it is a key ingredient in all sorts of recipes, from a quick snack to a really good meal.

½ cup salted macadamia nuts

1 Tbsp. coconut oil

1 tsp. minced garlic

2 Tbsp. diced red onion

1 tsp. minced ginger

¼ tsp. coriander

¼ tsp. cumin powder

½ cup coconut milk

¼ cup maple syrup

1 Tbsp. soy sauce

¼ tsp. chili flakes (optional)

½ cup salted creamy peanut butter

¼ cup lime juice

1 Dry toast the macadamia nuts in a pan over medium-high heat until they are golden brown. Set them aside.

2 Heat coconut oil in the pan, add the garlic, onion, ginger, coriander, and cumin, and sauté until the onion is soft, about 2–3 minutes.

3 Add the coconut milk, maple syrup, soy sauce, and chili flakes if you want spice. Cook for another 2–3 minutes.

4 Place toasted macadamia nuts, coconut milk mixture, peanut butter, and lime juice in a high-powered blender and blitz until smooth.

5 Serve over Summer Rolls (page 103), salad, rice, or just about any Asian-inspired meal that you like!

6 Store in an airtight container in the refrigerator for up to 1 week.

Oaxaca Mole Sauce

MAKES ABOUT 2½ CUPS

Sauce is everything in cooking. If the seasoning and sauce aren't right, then the whole dish will fall apart. Our Oaxaca Mole Sauce will hold all sorts of dishes together. We use it on tamales, tacos, burritos, and scrambled tofu. It'll add a delicious Mexican flavor to whatever your heart desires. It is tangy, spicy, creamy, and oh so good!

2 Tbsp. coconut oil

1 chile de arbol

½ guajillo pepper

1 pasilla pepper

¼ cup sesame seeds

¼ cup pumpkin seeds

4 allspice berries

2 bay leaves

2 cups chopped tomatillos

1 cup chopped tomato

1½ tsp. Himalayan pink salt

1 cup water

1 Heat the coconut oil in a medium-size skillet over medium heat. Place the arbol, guajillo, and pasilla peppers in the pan and sauté for 2–3 minutes.

2 Add sesame seeds, pumpkin seeds, allspice berries, and bay leaves and sauté for another 2 minutes.

3 Add the tomatillos, tomato, and salt and cook for an additional 1–2 minutes. Then stir in the water and let the mixture simmer for 3–5 minutes, or until the tomatillos are tender.

4 Pour the mixture into a high-powered blender and blitz for 45 seconds, or until smooth and creamy.

5 Place in an airtight container or squeeze bottle and refrigerate.

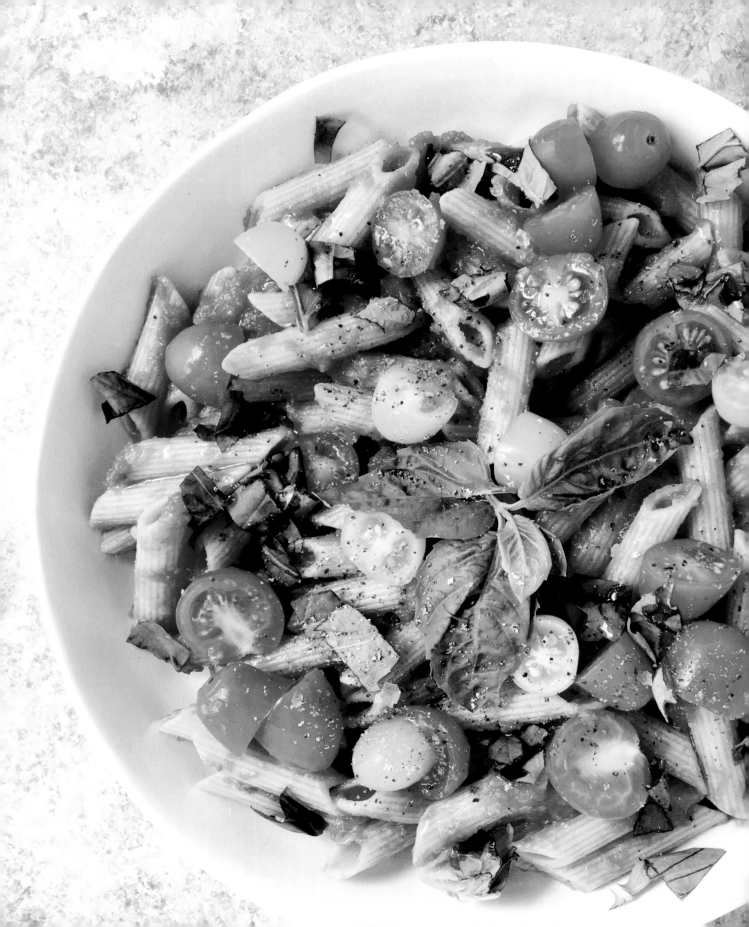

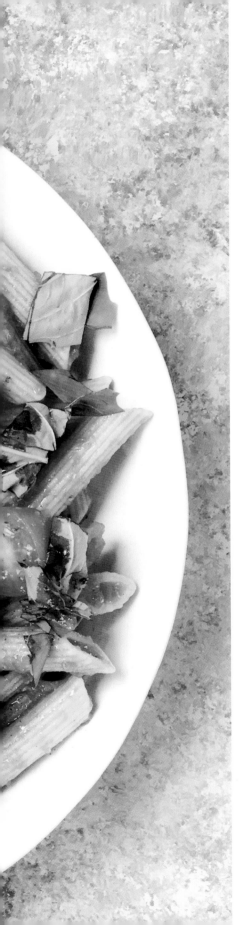

Sun-Dried Garden Marinara

MAKES 4 CUPS

Let's face it: marinara is one of the most well-received sauces in the world. Everyone loves its sweet, tangy, acidic, salty goodness and how it spices up pasta, pizza, and many other dishes. Our homemade recipe was complicated at first. We blanched garden tomatoes and used fresh herbs from scratch, and the process was labor intensive. The only thing that could have made it more complicated would have been moving to Italy, buying a plot of land, and starting our own tomato and herb garden! So we sat down and figured out how to make it more accessible. The end result: a smooth, beautiful sauce that hits all the right points but can be easily prepared even if you are living a hectic life full of work, kids, and obligations.

1 cup sun-dried tomatoes

5 large, ripe garden tomatoes of your choice

At least 5 garlic cloves, unpeeled, plus 1 Tbsp. minced garlic

5 Tbsp. olive oil

1 tsp. Himalayan pink salt

¼ tsp. pepper

1 large stem fresh rosemary, leaves still on

½ cup diced red onion

¼ tsp. thyme

1 tsp. oregano

2 Tbsp. chopped fresh basil

1 Tbsp. maple syrup

▶

Sun-Dried Garden Marinara *(cont.)*

1 Preheat the oven to 450 degrees F.

2 Soak the sun-dried tomatoes in 2 cups of warm water for 1 hour.

3 While the sun-dried tomatoes soak, wash the garden tomatoes, then make a small X in the bottom of each tomato using the point of a knife. Place the garden tomatoes on a large baking sheet with the X facing up.

4 Crush 5 cloves of garlic and place over the tomatoes with the peel still around the cloves. Pour 2 Tbsp. of the olive oil over the tomatoes, then sprinkle with ½ tsp. of the salt, followed by all the pepper. Lastly, place the rosemary stem across the tops of the tomatoes.

5 Place tomatoes in the oven and bake for 25–30 minutes. The garlic peels and rosemary should burn a little to infuse the tomatoes with flavor and aromas.

6 Remove the tomatoes from the oven, peel the garlic, and discard the garlic peels and rosemary stem. Peel the skins off the tomatoes and cut off the rough ends if needed.

7 Place the peeled tomatoes and garlic in a high-powered blender and set aside without blending.

8 Heat a large frying pan and stir in the remaining 3 Tbsp. of olive oil, diced red onion, 1 Tbsp. minced garlic, thyme, and oregano. Sauté over medium-low heat until the onions and garlic are soft.

9 Drain the sun-dried tomatoes, add them to the onions, and cook for another 3–5 minutes to soften.

10 Add the sautéed vegetables to the oven-baked tomatoes in the blender, along with the fresh basil, maple syrup, and remaining salt. Blend until smooth. Adjust the salt according to taste.

Avocado Mint Chutney

MAKES ABOUT 1 CUP

Mint chutney is a staple in Indian cuisine. Our family loves this variation, and we use it on salads, Samosa Pot Pie (page 153), and just about anything that needs some sauce. It is healthy, light, and scrumptious!

1 packed cup destemmed fresh mint

1 packed cup chopped fresh cilantro

2 Tbsp. maple syrup

¾ tsp. Himalayan pink salt

1 cup water

½ cup chopped avocado

¼ cup chopped red onion

2 Tbsp. lime juice

Pinch of chili powder

1 Place all the ingredients in a high-powered blender or food processor and blitz for 45 seconds, or until smooth.

2 Store in an airtight container in the refrigerator for up to 1 week.

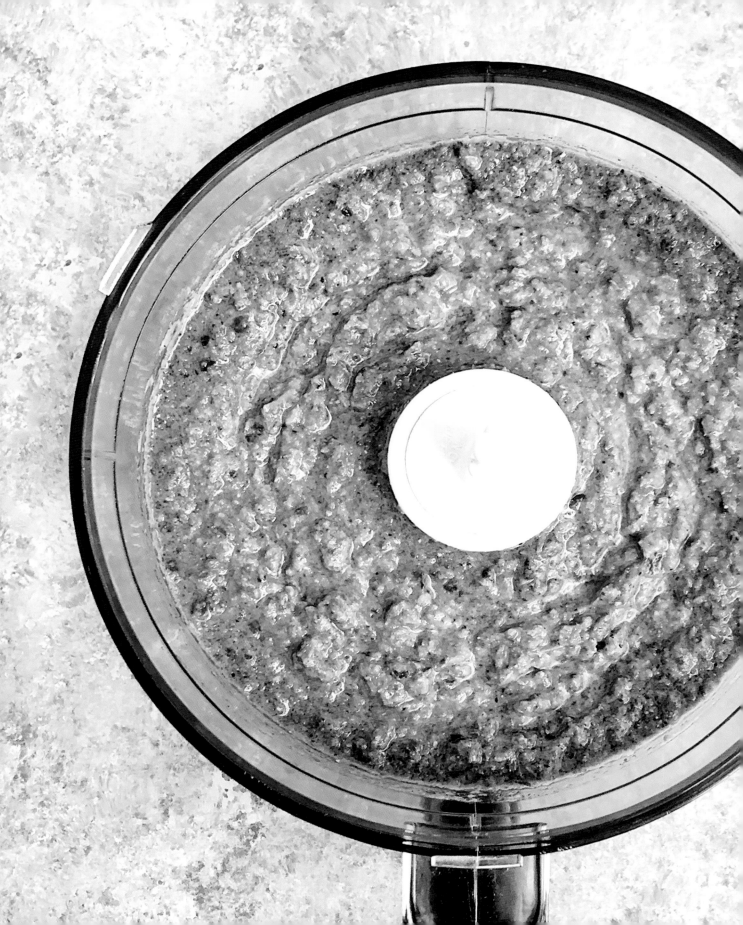

Fresh and Creamy Pesto

MAKES 1½ CUPS

Pesto is one of our favorite things to make, and you will be surprised at how fast and easy it is to prepare. This mighty pesto sauce will completely transform a bowl of pasta with that extra kick of flavor and goodness. It is packed with healthy omegas and vitamin E. The spinach and basil are an excellent source of vitamin K and are loaded with fiber. We love it so much that we use it for more than pasta. You can spread it on sandwiches, add it to veggie hummus wraps, or serve it in a bowl as a dip for crackers. Sometimes we even use it instead of tomato sauce on a pizza crust. We like the recipe below, but feel free to mix it up and throw in hemp seeds or different greens, like parsley or kale. Yum-yum!

2 garlic cloves, peeled

½ cup walnuts

½ cup pine nuts

1½ cups basil

1 cup spinach

⅓ cup olive oil

¼ cup nutritional yeast

½ tsp. Himalayan pink salt

1 In a food processor, pulse the garlic cloves until finely minced.

2 Add the walnuts and pine nuts and pulse again.

3 Next, add the basil, spinach, and olive oil and pulse until smooth. You will have to stop a few times and scrape down the sides with a spatula. If the mixture is too thick, try adding 1 Tbsp. of additional olive oil or water.

4 Lastly, pour in the nutritional yeast and salt and process until smooth.

5 Add to your favorite pasta and indulge!

Cashew Cream Everything Sauce

MAKES ABOUT 2 CUPS

Our family loves this sauce and we literally put it on everything—hence the name. We cover nachos, rice bowls, baked potatoes, tacos, and so much more with it. It's full of healthy fats, antioxidants, vitamins, and minerals, and it can brighten up just about any dish you make with an extra dash of flavor. You will want to keep a bottle of this in your fridge at all times. (It keeps well for up to one week.) We keep ours in a squeeze bottle with a small tip so we can make fun designs over our food.

2 cups raw cashews, soaked for at least 2–3 hours

1½ cups water

½ cup fresh lemon juice

1 tsp. Himalayan pink salt

½ tsp. garlic powder

1 Place all the ingredients in a high-powered blender and blitz for 45 seconds. Stop, then blitz for another 45 seconds, or until creamy smooth.

Mango Salsa

MAKES ABOUT 3 CUPS

This simple and quick yet colorful salsa is one of our favorites to make on taco night. We are not sure about you, but our family is *really big* on taco night. In fact, we often have it more than once a week. The sweetness from the mango gives the salsa that extra boost of flavor, contrasting with the salty. This beautiful salsa is so fun and festive, you can toss it on top of nachos, salads, or even an open avocado half. It's sooooo good!

2–3 mangos, peeled, pitted, and diced, or 2 cups frozen diced mango, thawed

1 cup diced tomato

½ small red onion, finely chopped

½ cup chopped cilantro

½ jalapeño pepper, chopped (more if you like spicy)

2 limes

Salt to taste

1 Toss all ingredients except the limes together in a bowl. Squeeze the juice from the limes over the top. Toss again.

2 Add salt to taste and serve.

How to dice a mango:

1 *Find the stem and cut vertically down each side of it. Peel fruit apart into two halves.*

2 *With a paring knife, cut a grid pattern into the flesh of each half. Be careful not to cut through the skin.*

3 *With a large spoon, scoop the cut fruit from the mango skin.*

Cashew Parmesan Cheese

MAKES 1 CUP

This Cashew Parmesan Cheese has a permanent spot in our fridge. We replace it as soon as it runs out. It is the perfect final touch to all sorts of dishes. We sprinkle it on top of salads, soups, pastas, and more. All you need is 30 seconds to make this—not bad for a dairy-free alternative that tastes great and is super nutritious! Our Cashew Parmesan Cheese is loaded with healthy fats, fiber, vitamin B12, vitamin E, vitamin K, zinc, magnesium, plus a whole lot more. Try this and change your cheese life forever!

1 cup raw cashews

1 garlic clove, peeled

1 Tbsp. nutritional yeast

¼ tsp. Himalayan pink salt

1 Place all the ingredients in a high-speed blender and process until it resembles Parmesan cheese. Do not overprocess, or you will release the oils from the cashews and end up with cashew butter.

2 Store in an airtight glass container and keep in the refrigerator for up to 1 week.

You can easily interchange the cashews with other nuts, such as pecans, walnuts, and almonds, or with seeds, such as sunflower seeds and pumpkin seeds.

Miso Ginger Dressing

MAKES 1 CUP

Dressing is the key to any salad. It is the paint to a canvas, an instrument in a musician's hand. It's that spark that makes us say yay or nay to a bowlful of greens! This dressing is wonderful on a cold soba noodle salad or any Asian-inspired dish. We also use this as a dipping sauce.

2 Tbsp. finely minced ginger

3 Tbsp. sesame oil

¼ cup maple syrup

1 Tbsp. miso

1 tsp. minced garlic

¼ cup soy sauce

¼ cup vinegar

⅓ cup plus 2 Tbsp. olive oil

1 Place all the ingredients in a high-powered blender and mix until smooth. We like to turn the blender on high for 45 seconds twice.

2 Pour into a plastic squeeze bottle or a jar and refrigerate for up to 1 week.

Creamy Vegan Ranch

MAKES ABOUT 1½ CUPS

Get your veggies out and say hello to your new favorite dip! This creamy nondairy ranch is a guilt-free pleasure you can enjoy any time of day. Made with cashews for the creamy texture, it is bursting with healthy fats, fiber, and vitamin B12, along with other vitamins and minerals, such as zinc, magnesium, and vitamin E. This versatile sauce doubles as a dip, so you can pair it with fresh veggies, spread it on a sandwich, dollop it onto a taco, or simply pour it on your favorite salad.

1 cup soaked raw cashews

¾ cup water or unsweetened almond milk

2 Tbsp. fresh lemon juice

1½ Tbsp. apple cider vinegar

1 Tbsp. fresh dill

¼ cup nutritional yeast

1 tsp. garlic powder

1 tsp. onion powder

½ tsp. Himalayan pink salt

1   Place all the ingredients into a high-speed blender and process until smooth and creamy. If you want a thinner consistency, add 1 Tbsp. of water at a time until you reach the desired result.

If you are using almond milk, make sure it is the plain, unsweetened kind and not vanilla flavored.

Shiitake Holiday Gravy

MAKES 2 CUPS

Gravy pairs so well with mashed potatoes it tastes like a combo that is meant to be. It's like the marriage of chocolate and peanut butter or salsa and tacos. Gravy amplifies the taste and creaminess of the potatoes and will add a boost of flavor to everything else on a holiday plate. The trick is to make it so that it is perfectly balanced. This Shiitake Holiday Gravy is a special variation we made just for Victoria, who doesn't like her gravy too oily, salty, or heavy. It is delicate and delicious, packed with flavor and smooth as can be. Plus it is high in protein. Victoria requests it every Thanksgiving now and always goes back for seconds!

1 tsp. grape-seed oil

1 cup minced shiitake mushrooms

2 Tbsp. plus ½ tsp. soy sauce

4 Tbsp. olive oil

4 Tbsp. garbanzo bean flour

2 cups water

1 In a small saucepan, heat the grape-seed oil over medium heat and toss in the minced shiitake mushrooms. Sauté, stirring, for 2–3 minutes, or until tender.

2 Stir in ½ tsp. soy sauce and turn off the heat. Set the mushrooms aside.

3 Pour the olive oil and garbanzo bean flour into a small pot and cook, stirring continuously, for 1–2 minutes.

4 Quickly stir in the remaining 2 Tbsp. soy sauce — you must work fast, or the mixture will stick — then stir in the water. Cook, stirring, over medium heat for 5–10 minutes, or until it thickens to a gravy consistency.

5 Turn off the heat when you have reached desired thickness. Stir in the mushrooms.

6 Serve over warm mashed potatoes and stuffing.

Whipped Cream from Heaven

MAKES 2 CUPS

This dish was a magical creation that took shape in one session. Usually recipe testing is a highly involved process that happens over time. This recipe, however, was a one-shot wonder that turned out utterly blissful. Loaded with good fats, vitamins, and minerals, it delivers a heavenly combination of flavor and goodness. It's a wonderful complement to all sorts of dishes. Pair it with pancakes, fresh berries, muffins, and cakes—anything you'd like to add a little extra heavenly love to!

1 cup soaked cashews

1 cup coconut cream, refrigerated overnight

2 Tbsp. maple syrup

½ cup coconut oil

1 Tbsp. sunflower lecithin

⅛ tsp. Himalayan pink salt

1 Place all the ingredients in a food processor or Vitamix and blend twice for 45 seconds each time, or until smooth.

2 Pour the resulting cream into a small glass or metal dish and place in the freezer for 30 minutes to set.

3 Take the cream out of the freezer and let it sit in the refrigerator for at least 1 hour before serving.

4 Store for about 2 weeks in the refrigerator.

Serve over a fresh bowl of berries or on top of our American Apple Pie (page 209).

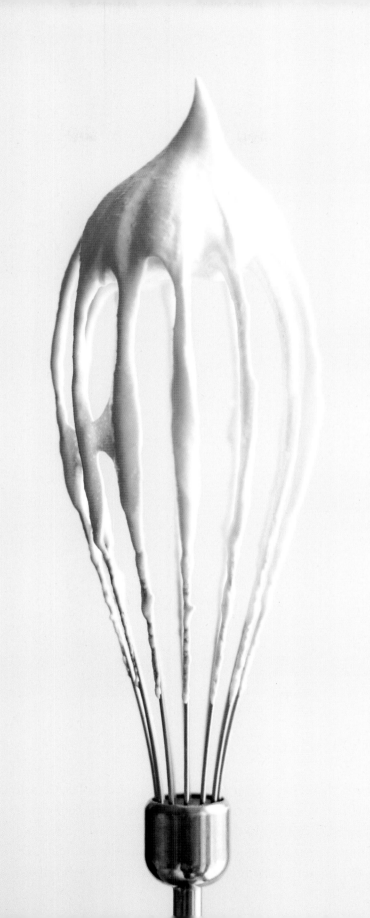

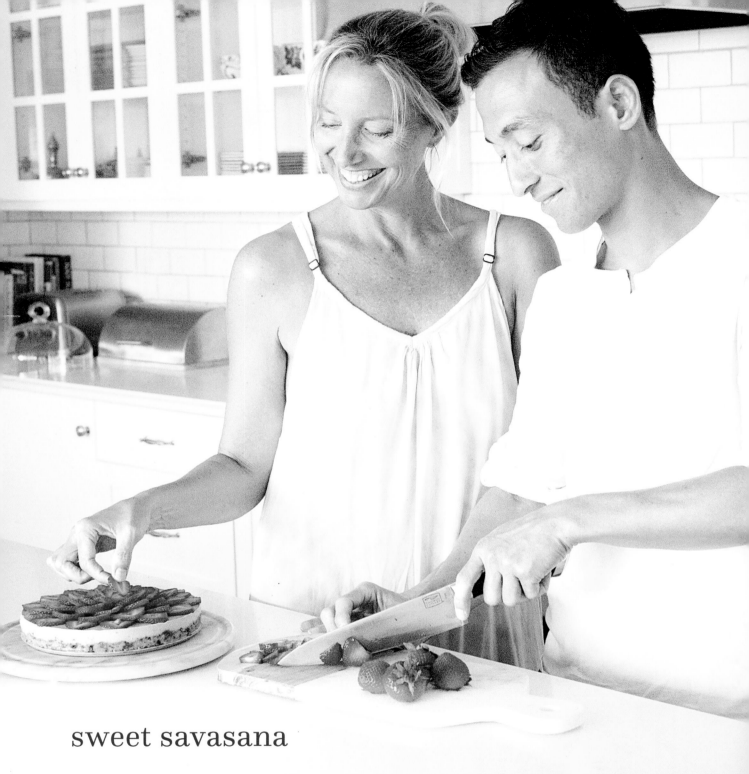

sweet savasana

The best part of a yoga class is at the very end, when the entire class lays down in *Savasana*, or Resting Pose. The hard work has been done, and we can completely let go and dive deep into restoration. Savasana is like dessert. Not only is it delicious, but it's also highly beneficial for managing stress hormones and anxiety and for restoring fatigued muscles. Similarly, our desserts not only taste incredible but also are packed full of essential nutrients.

desserts

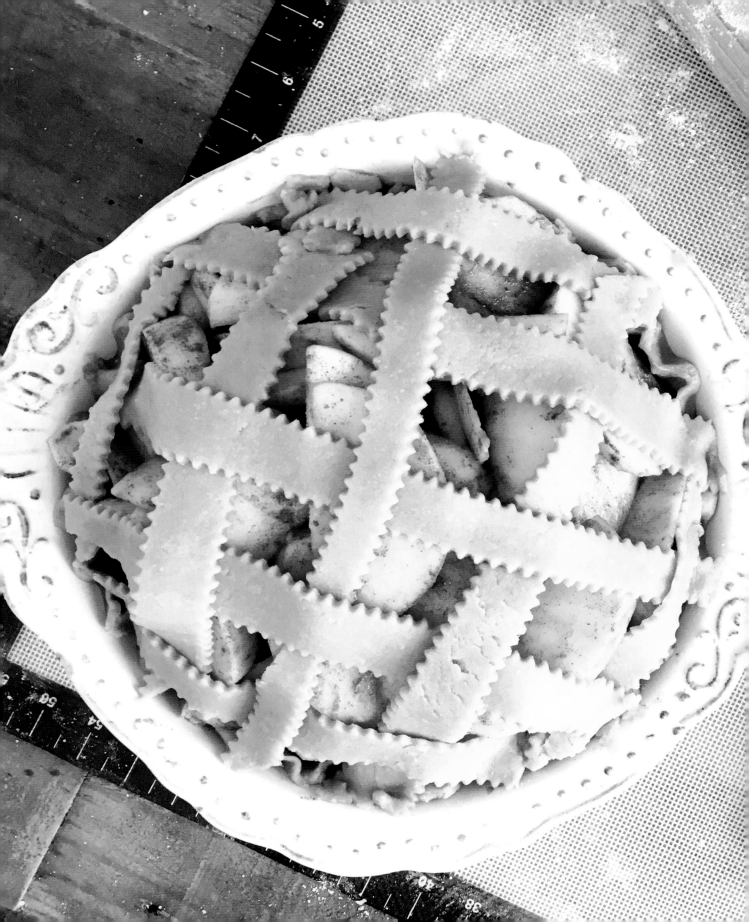

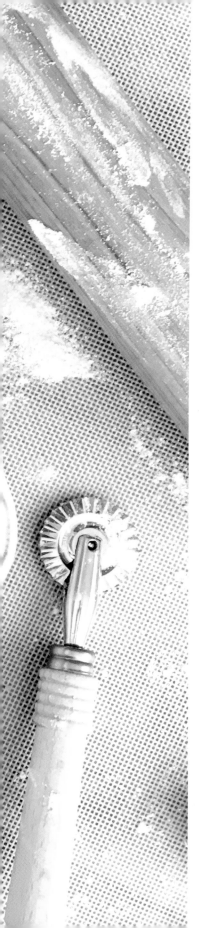

American Apple Pie

MAKES ONE 9-INCH PIE

Is there anything better than the smell of a fresh, homemade apple pie baking in your oven? We don't think so! This pie will fill your house with crisp apple and cozy cinnamon aromas. Don't be surprised if your neighbors knock on the door, hoping for a slice or two. It's that inviting. The crust is quick and simple to make, and you'll be amazed at how flaky it tastes without the dairy. The white whole-wheat pastry flour is light, feathery, and full of vitamins and minerals (unlike all-purpose white flour). The apples are bursting with healthy nutrition, such as antioxidants, fiber, and vitamin C. This pie is so full of goodness you can have it for breakfast.

For the crust

2 cups white whole-wheat pastry flour

1 tsp. Himalayan pink salt

1 Tbsp. coconut sugar

½ cup coconut oil

½ cup ice-cold water

1 Preheat the oven to 350 degrees F.

2 Place all of the piecrust ingredients in a food processor and blend. The mixture will form a large ball of dough in no time at all. Set aside one-quarter of the dough for the crisscross topping.

3 Lightly sprinkle your clean work surface and a rolling pin with flour. Roll the larger portion of the dough into a large circle, about 12 inches in diameter. Transfer the circle to a 9-inch pie pan. Create a ridge around the rim with your fingers. Then poke holes in the bottom of the dough with a fork. This will help the piecrust bake evenly.

4 Set aside in the refrigerator and prepare the filling.

▶

American Apple Pie (*cont.*)

For the filling

5–6 organic apples

½–¾ cup maple syrup

1 tsp. cinnamon

3 Tbsp. white whole-wheat
pastry flour

1   Peel and core the apples and slice into thin pieces.

2   Place the apple slices in a large bowl and add the remaining ingredients. Stir to mix thoroughly.

3   Remove the crust from the fridge and pour the apple mixture into it.

4   Roll out the remaining dough and cut into 1-inch strips. Weave the strips in a crisscross fashion on top of the filling. Secure the edges to the side of the pie by pinching them together with the bottom part of the crust.

5   Bake the pie in the oven for 45 minutes to 1 hour. You can check the apples with a fork—they are done when they feel tender—and the lattice top should be golden brown.

6   Remove the pie from the oven and let it sit for about 15 minutes, to allow the liquid to thicken and cool.

Rawsome Carrot Cake

This is a refreshing and light take on a classic dessert. It offers all of the flavor and that wonderful complexity that you'd find in a standard carrot cake, but without the sugary heaviness. Rawsome Carrot Cake won't leave you tired. On the contrary—it'll make you feel refreshed. This recipe has such clean ingredients that when we eat it for breakfast, it gives us energy for the day!

For the cake base

2 cups walnuts

½ cup oat flour

½ cup unsweetened desiccated coconut

½ cup coconut flour

½ cup melted coconut oil

2 Tbsp. lemon juice

2 tsp. vanilla extract

2 tsp. cinnamon

1 tsp. ground ginger

½ tsp. ground nutmeg

2 tsp. lemon zest

2 cups pitted dates (preferably Medjool)

Pinch of Himalayan pink salt

2 cups finely grated carrots

1. Place walnuts in a food processor and blitz until they are reduced to fine granules. Add the oat flour, desiccated coconut, coconut flour, coconut oil, lemon juice, vanilla extract, cinnamon, ginger, nutmeg, lemon zest, dates, and salt and blitz until a cake-like batter forms.

2. Fold the grated carrrots into the batter with your hands or a spatula.

3. Pour the carrot cake batter in a nonstick 9-inch cheesecake pan and pat down with your hands so the top is smooth and even. You can lightly grease your with hands with coconut oil to prevent the batter from sticking to them.

4. Set the cake base in the freezer while you make the icing.

▶

Rawsome Carrot Cake *(cont.)*

For the icing

2 cups soaked raw cashews

½ cup unsweetened coconut milk

½ cup melted coconut oil

6 Tbsp. maple syrup

4 Tbsp. lemon juice

1 tsp. vanilla extract

Pinch Himalayan pink salt

1 tsp. lemon zest

1 Place all the icing ingredients in a blender and blitz twice for 45 seconds each time, or until very smooth.

2 Remove the raw cake batter from the freezer. Pour the icing on top and smooth it out with the back of a spoon or a spatula.

3 Return the cake to the freezer for 1 hour to set. Then you can transfer it to the refrigerator to keep cool until you serve it.

Victoria likes to use a chocolate shaver to shred the carrots, as it produces a finer grain and is a better tool than a normal grater. However, a normal grater will work fine.

The Ultimate Chocolate Cake

MAKES ONE 8-INCH ROUND LAYER CAKE

The Ultimate Chocolate Cake is one of the most ridiculously moist, melt-in-your-mouth, drool-over desserts we have ever eaten. It's perfect for any occasion, or let it serve as a celebration unto itself! Certainly, eating something so delicious without feeling guilty is cause to celebrate. Made from whole grains, healthy sweeteners, and nourishing fats, this is one treat that you can happily enjoy as many servings of as you like. So what are you waiting for? Let's get in the kitchen and start baking!

For the cake base

1⅔ cups white whole-wheat pastry flour

½ cup unsweetened cocoa powder

1 tsp. baking soda

½ tsp. Himalayan pink salt

1 cup maple syrup

1¼ cups water

⅓ cup melted coconut oil

1 tsp. white or apple cider vinegar

½ tsp. vanilla extract

1. Preheat the oven to 325 degrees F. Make sure your rack is in the center of the oven.

2. Lightly oil and flour two 8-inch cake pans with coconut oil and about 1 Tbsp. flour. Pat the outside of the pans upside-down to remove excess flour. Set aside.

3. In a large mixing bowl, sift together the flour, cocoa powder, baking soda, and salt.

4. In a separate bowl, stir together the maple syrup, water, coconut oil, vinegar, and vanilla extract.

5. Stir together the wet and dry ingredients just to combine. *Do not overmix.*

6. Fill each cake pan with batter about halfway. Bake for 20 minutes.

7. Remove from the oven and let cool for about 15–20 minutes while you prepare the icing.

▶

The Ultimate Chocolate Cake (*cont.*)

For the Homemade Powdered Sugar

1 cup coconut sugar

2 Tbsp. cornstarch

1 Blend ingredients in a high-powered blender for 45 seconds, until powdered.

For the Chocolate Almond Butter Icing

1¼ cups Homemade
Powdered Sugar

2 Tbsp. vegan butter

2 Tbsp. unsweetened nondairy milk

1 Tbsp. creamy almond butter

½ tsp. vanilla extract

1 In a medium-size mixing bowl, combine 1¼ cups Homemade Powdered Sugar, vegan butter, nondairy milk, almond butter, and vanilla extract. Blend with a hand mixer for about 3–5 minutes, or until a thick, gooey frosting forms.

2 Immediately frost and assemble the cake or refrigerate the icing until ready to use.

Raw Lemon Raspberry Cheesecake

MAKES ONE 9-INCH CHEESECAKE

Treat your taste buds to an explosion of flavors with this Raw Lemon Raspberry Cheesecake. Loaded with healthy fats, fiber, vitamins, and minerals without sacrificing flavor, this is a win-win dessert recipe. Victoria often teaches this recipe in her cooking classes, because it's very simple to make. It also looks sensational as a centerpiece at a dinner party—the vibrant raspberry color really pops. If you are using frozen raspberries (which we use most often, unless it is raspberry season), don't forget to defrost them in their bag; they need to be at room temperature so they don't make the coconut oil clump. Give it a whirl and treat yourself!

For the crust

1 cup raw almonds

3 Tbsp. raw cacao powder

¾ cup pitted dates
(preferably Medjool)

Pinch of Himalayan pink salt

1   Place the almonds in a food processor and process until they are broken into small pieces.

2   Add the cacao powder, dates, and salt. Process until the mixture will hold together with gentle pressure. If it's not sticking together well enough, add 1 Tbsp. water at a time until it reaches the right consistency.

3   Grease a 9-inch pie pan or cheesecake pan with coconut oil and then press the mixture into the pan with your fingers.

For smaller, bite-sized versions, you can make these in a silicone muffin pan instead of a larger pan.

For the filling

2 cups soaked cashews

1 cup unsweetened almond milk

¾ cup maple syrup

¾ cup lemon juice

Zest from 2 lemons

1 Tbsp. vanilla extract

⅛ tsp. Himalayan pink salt

1 12-oz. bag frozen raspberries, thawed, or about 1 cup fresh

3 Tbsp. sunflower lecithin

¾ cup coconut oil

1 Place the soaked cashews and almond milk in a food processor and blend until creamy. Add maple syrup, lemon juice, lemon zest, vanilla extract, and salt. Process until creamy, 3–5 minutes.

2 Add the raspberries and process again until blended.

3 Add the sunflower lecithin and coconut oil. Process once more until smooth and creamy.

4 Pour the filling mixture into the prepared crust. Place in freezer for 1–2 hours to set. Remove from freezer and serve.

5 Cheesecake will keep for 4–5 days if stored covered in the refrigerator. It will last for 7–10 days in the freezer. We keep ours covered in the freezer and take it out 10–15 minutes before serving.

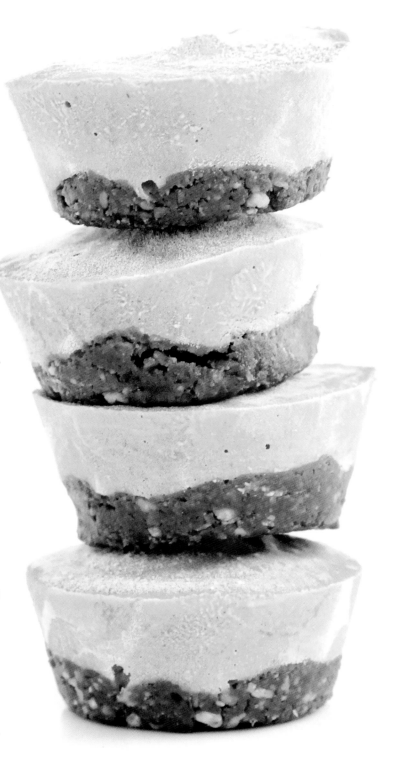

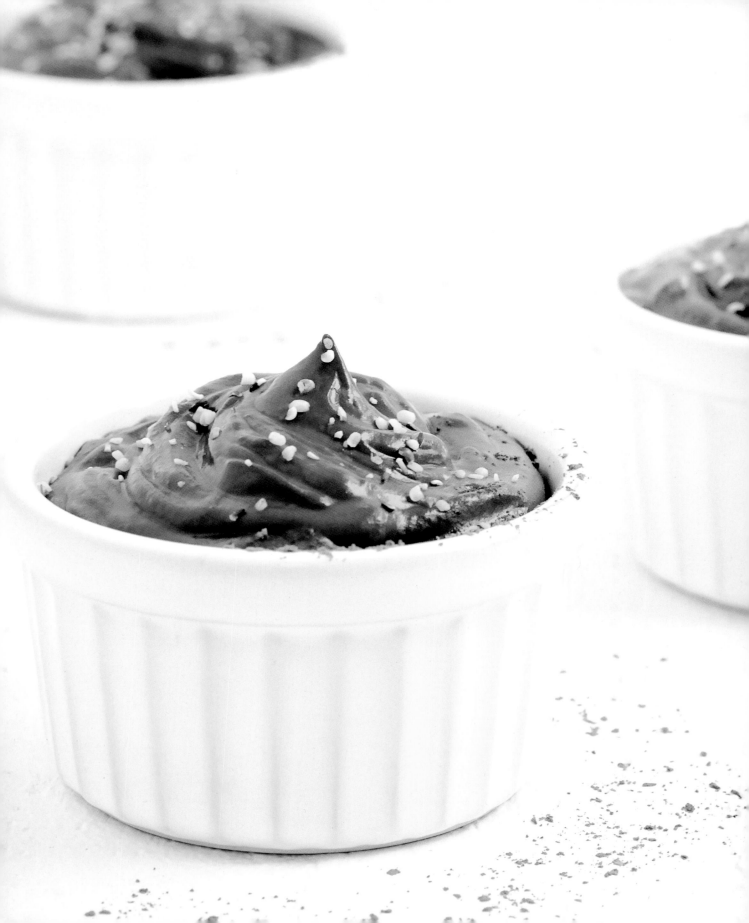

Creamy Chocolate Pudding

SERVES 4

You are never going to guess what secret ingredient this pudding contains: avocado! Your kids will never know it's there. I love making this pudding in the summer and dipping fresh strawberries from our local farmers' market in it. Blueberries and raspberries are great toppers, too, plus a little splash of hemp seeds. Or simply dice a banana on top. This pudding is raw, except for the maple syrup. It is packed full of healthy fats, antioxidants, and fiber. We would make a double batch if we were you!

½ cup maple syrup

½ cup raw cacao powder

2 large or 3 small ripe avocados, peeled and pitted

1 tsp. vanilla extract

½ cup water

Pinch of Himalayan pink salt

1 In a food processor, add the maple syrup, cacao powder, and avocados. Process until well combined.

2 Add the vanilla extract, water, and salt and process to get the desired consistency. The amount of processing time will vary according to the size of your avocados. The pudding should be creamy and completely smooth, so you might have to process longer than you think.

3 Chill for 30 minutes to 1 hour and serve.

4 Store in an airtight container in the fridge for 3–4 days.

Raw Chocolate Brownie Bites

MAKES 15–18 ONE-INCH BALLS

Need a chocolate fix? These bite-size brownies are the perfect snack for chocolate aficionados and novices alike. Made with raw walnuts, dates, and cacao powder, they are loaded with antioxidants, omega-3s, vitamin E, magnesium, iron, and fiber. You can enjoy them for breakfast, as a pre- or postworkout treat, for an afternoon snack, or as a dessert. Bring a batch to a dinner party and watch them disappear in seconds!

1½ cups walnuts

1½ cups pitted dates (preferably Medjool)

½ cup raw cacao powder

¼ tsp. Himalayan pink salt

1   Place the walnuts in a food processor and process until they become a fine flour.

2   Add the dates, cacao powder, and salt. Process until they form a sticky mixture.

3   Roll them into 1-inch bite-size balls or pat them into an 8x8-inch pan lined with parchment paper.

4   Store in an airtight container for up to 1 week (if they last that long!). They can be refrigerated or left on the countertop at room temperature.

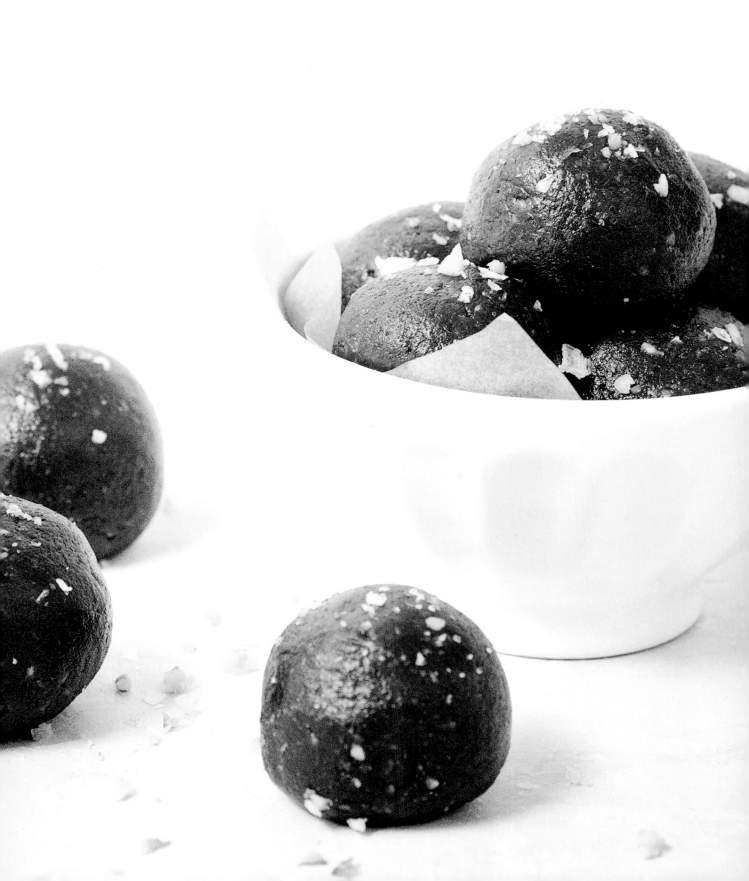

The Perfect Chocolate Chip Cookie

MAKES ABOUT 18 COOKIES

Chocolate chip cookies are an American classic. To many of us, they evoke memories of childhood—reaching into that cookie jar at a friend's house, our little legs dangling from the chair, not quite long enough to reach the floor. Or standing at a kitchen counter, wooden spoon in hand, stirring the mixture with a loved one by our side. You don't need to miss out on this nostalgic treat. We've come up with a healthy version, replacing the white flour and white sugar with more wholesome ingredients. We guarantee these cookies will be loved by people of all ages. Give them a try and remember to share the love!

1½ cups white whole-wheat pastry flour

1 tsp. baking soda

½ tsp. baking powder

½ tsp. Himalayan pink salt

½ cup melted coconut oil

½ cup brown sugar

¼ cup organic cane sugar

¼ cup unsweetened almond milk

1 flax egg (page 56)

½ cup vegan chocolate chips

1   Preheat the oven to 350 degrees F. Line two medium-size baking sheets with parchment paper.

2   In a large mixing bowl, sift together the flour, baking soda, and baking powder until well combined. Stir in the salt.

3   Pour in the melted coconut oil and mix thoroughly.

4   Next, add in the brown sugar, cane sugar, almond milk, and flax egg and blend with a hand mixer until well combined. Fold in the chocolate chips.

5   Form the dough into 1-inch balls and place on the parchment paper-lined baking sheets, leaving plenty of room in between the balls.

6   Bake for 15 minutes, then let the cookies cool for at least 5–7 minutes before moving them to a cooling rack.

7   Store in an airtight container.

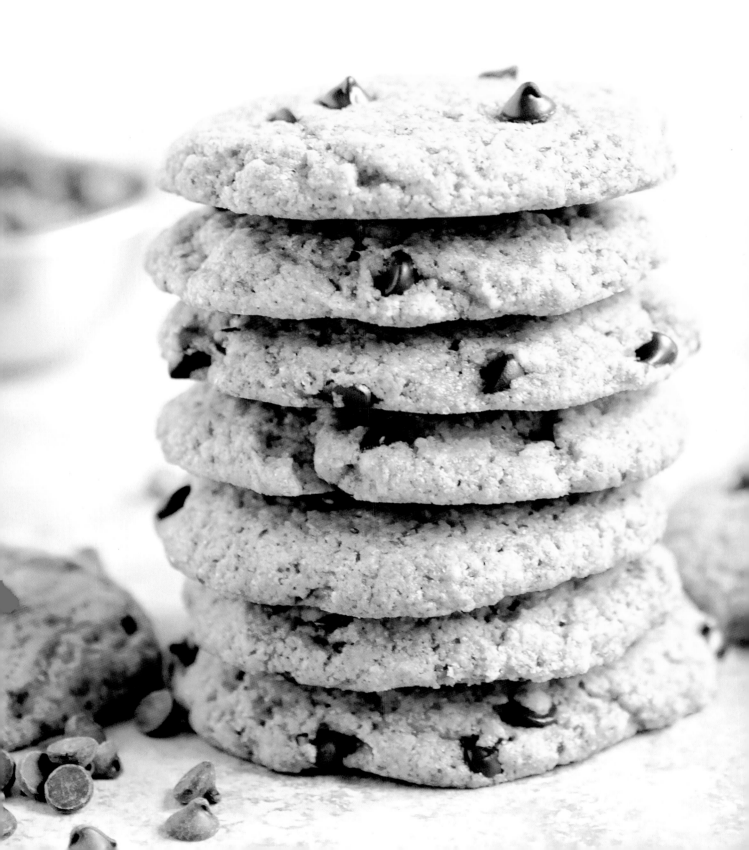

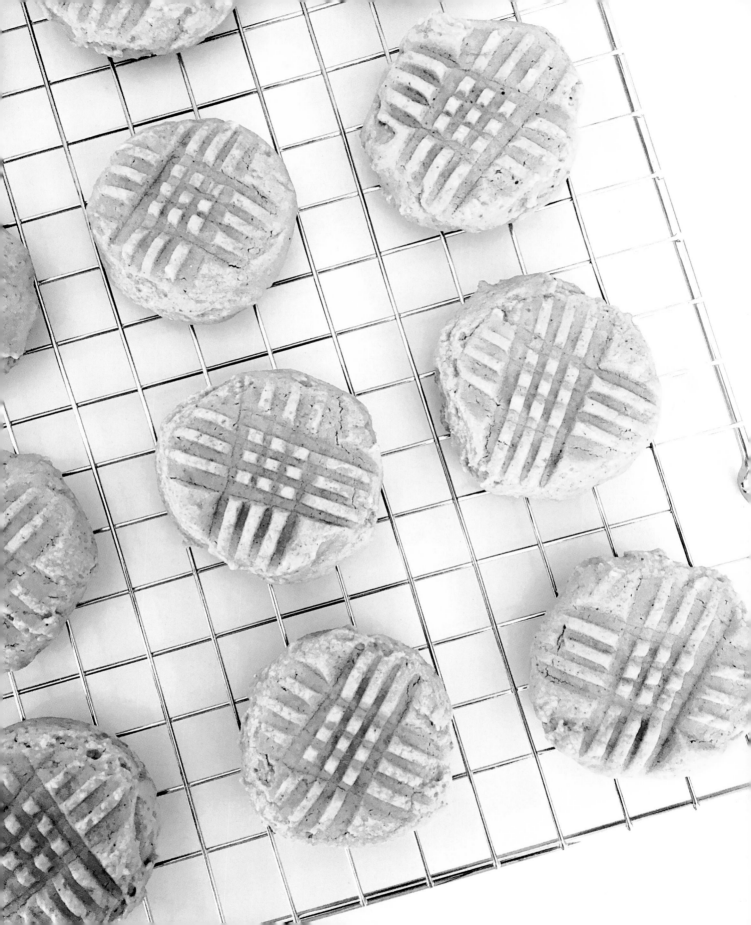

Guilt-Free, Gluten-Free Peanut Butter Cookies

MAKES 1 DOZEN

These melt-in-your-mouth, soft, chewy peanut butter cookies will have you hooked from the first bite. A perennial favorite in our house, this recipe is often doubled because we love it so much. It's a wholesome treat that appeals to adults and children alike. We offer these cookies to our son and his friends as an after-school snack. Sometimes we make ice cream sandwiches with them, putting a small scoop of vanilla or chocolate vegan ice cream in between two cookies. Yum!

1¼ cups brown rice flour

½ tsp. baking soda

½ tsp. Himalayan pink salt

½ cup organic creamy peanut butter

½ cup maple syrup

¼ cup olive oil

½ tsp. vanilla extract

1　Preheat the oven to 350 degrees F. Line a medium-size baking sheet with parchment paper.

2　In a medium bowl, stir the flour, baking soda, and salt together.

3　In a separate bowl stir together the peanut butter, maple syrup, olive oil, and vanilla extract. Make sure your peanut butter is soft and almost runny to start. If it's not, warm it up in a pan first until it softens up.

4　Pour the flour mixture over the peanut butter mixture and stir until barely combined. It will still look a bit dusty. Let the dough sit for 5 minutes, and then give it one more quick stir.

5　Drop the dough by heaping tablespoons onto the parchment paper-lined baking sheet. Gently press down on each one with the back of a fork to get a crisscross effect. If your fork sticks to the dough, just run it under hot water before each crisscross.

6　Bake for 10 minutes. Let the cookies cool for 10 minutes before removing them from the baking sheet.

If you do not have brown rice flour, you can substitute whole-wheat, spelt, and/or oat flour. All will work in this recipe. Just remember that if you use whole-wheat or spelt, the cookies will not be gluten free.

Sweet and Salty Bites

MAKES 10–15 ONE-INCH BALLS

These Sweet and Salty Bites are filled with a burst of flavors. First, think chocolate chip cookie dough. Sweetness from dates and chocolate chips. Then, there's a perfect contrast of saltiness from cashews and Himalayan pink salt. The best of both worlds! The dates provide steady energy, and the cashews are rich in vitamin E, magnesium, and zinc. A perfect snack!

1½ cups raw cashews

1½ cups pitted dates (preferably Medjool)

½ cup vegan chocolate chips

½ tsp. Himalayan pink salt

2 tsp. vanilla extract

1 Tbsp. water

1 Pulse the cashews in a food processor until they are reduced to a fine flour. Add the dates, chocolate chips, salt, vanilla extract, and water and pulse again until all the ingredients stick together. You may need to stop and scrape down the sides with a spatula.

2 Roll the mixture into bite-size balls and set them on a serving plate.

3 Refrigerate for about 30 minutes. Remove from the fridge and serve.

4 Store in an airtight container for up to 1 week (if they last that long!).

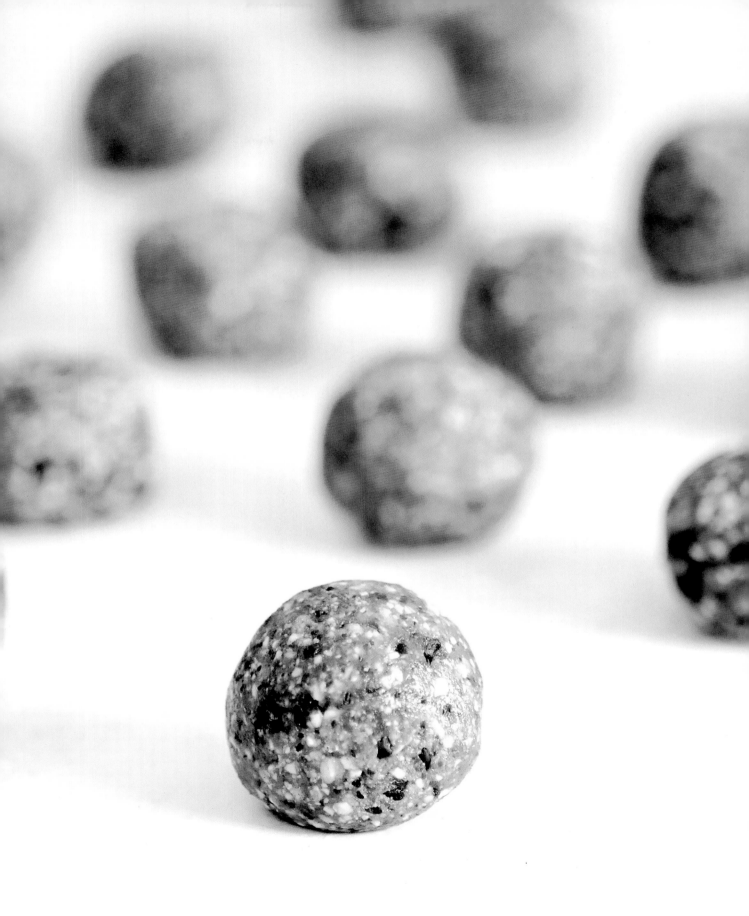

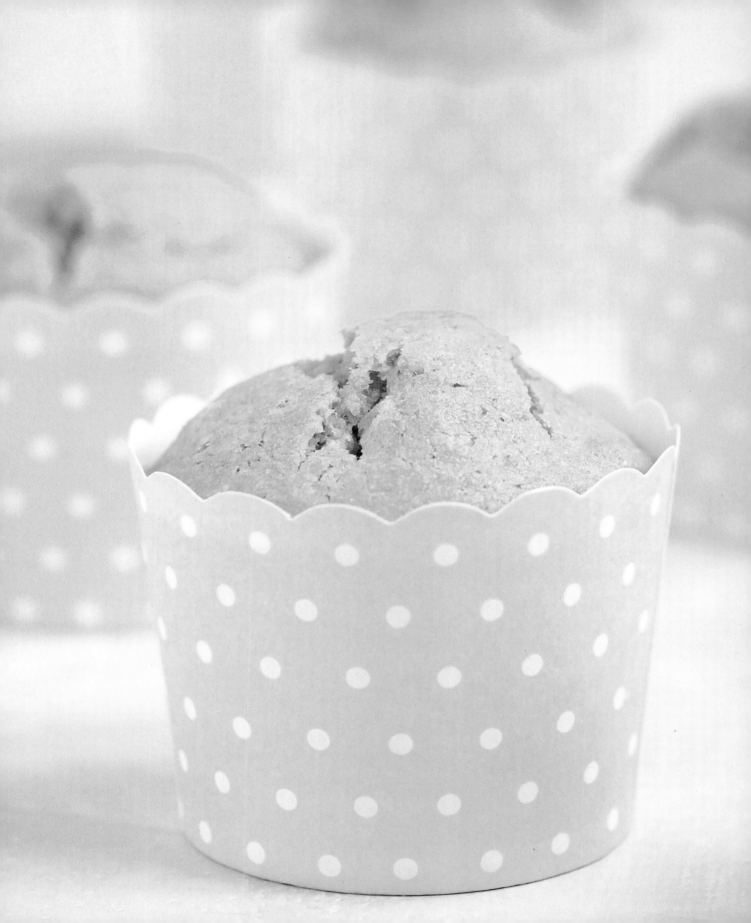

The Vanilla Cupcake

MAKES 1 DOZEN

When our son was very small, he loved vanilla cake. He wanted "vanilla everything" on his birthday. So we've tested out all sorts of vanilla cake recipes. This one is the best of them all. We turned it into a cupcake recipe, because kids love cupcakes. (See the tip below for the cake version.) These are moist and fluffy, and—even if your kids don't believe it—they're very healthy. They're grown-up approved, too. Happy baking!

1¾ cups white whole-wheat pastry flour

1 tsp. baking soda

½ tsp. Himalayan pink salt

¾ cup maple syrup

1 cup unsweetened almond milk

⅓ cup olive oil

1 Tbsp. apple cider vinegar

2 tsp. vanilla extract

1   Preheat the oven to 350 degrees F. Line a muffin tin with paper liners or coat with coconut or olive oil.

2   In a large bowl, sift the flour to get rid of any clumps. Mix the flour with baking soda and salt.

3   In a separate bowl, mix together the maple syrup, almond milk, olive oil, apple cider vinegar, and vanilla extract.

4   Pour the wet ingredients into the dry ingredients and stir just to mix. Do not overmix, or your cake will be too chewy.

5   Pour the batter into the muffin cups. Bake in the oven for 28 minutes, rotating the pan after 14 minutes.

6   Let cool for at least 10–15 minutes before serving.

If you are making this into a cake, oil and flour a 9-inch round pan. Pour the batter into the pan until it is half-filled—no more than that. Bake the cake for 30 minutes on the middle rack of your oven.

Brown Rice Crispy Treats

MAKES 9–12 BARS

A chewy, gooey Rice Krispies Treat is mouthwateringly delicious. We've come up with a heavenly alternative that is just as tasty *and* guilt free! Whole-grain brown rice, almond butter, and maple syrup are the main ingredients, and together they provide healthy fats and fiber, along with all sorts of vitamins and minerals, including calcium, copper, magnesium, and vitamin E. Whether you're indulging on your own or sharing with family and friends, you'll be reaching for more—and why not?

½ cup almond butter

⅓ cup maple syrup

1 tsp. vanilla extract

3 cups brown rice cereal, such as One Degree

1 Line the bottom and sides of a 9x9 baking pan with parchment paper. We like to cut two pieces of parchment paper and lay one down in each direction so the paper doesn't bunch up in the corners.

2 In a small pot over medium to low heat, stir and melt the almond butter, maple syrup, and vanilla extract together for 30 seconds to 1 minute, until the mixture is soft and blended.

3 Turn off the heat. Add the brown rice cereal and stir together until the cereal is thoroughly coated in the almond butter mixture.

4 Pour the rice crispy goo into the parchment paper-lined pan. Use another piece of parchment paper to help you press the mixture evenly into the pan with your hands. The paper will prevent the mixture from sticking to your fingers.

5 Chill the treats in your fridge for 30 minutes. Cut into pieces and serve.

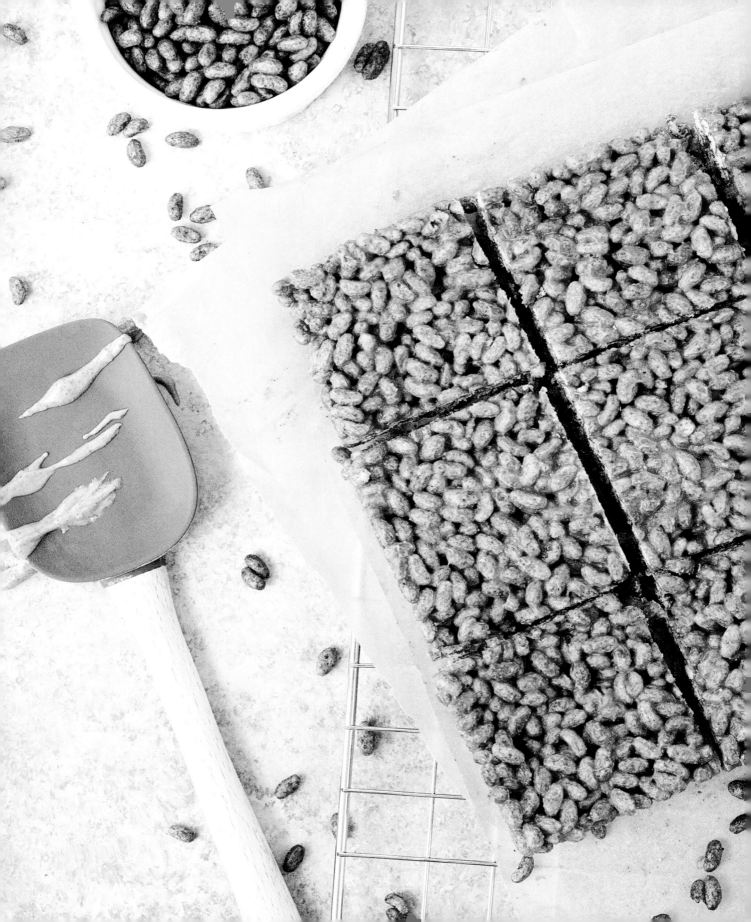

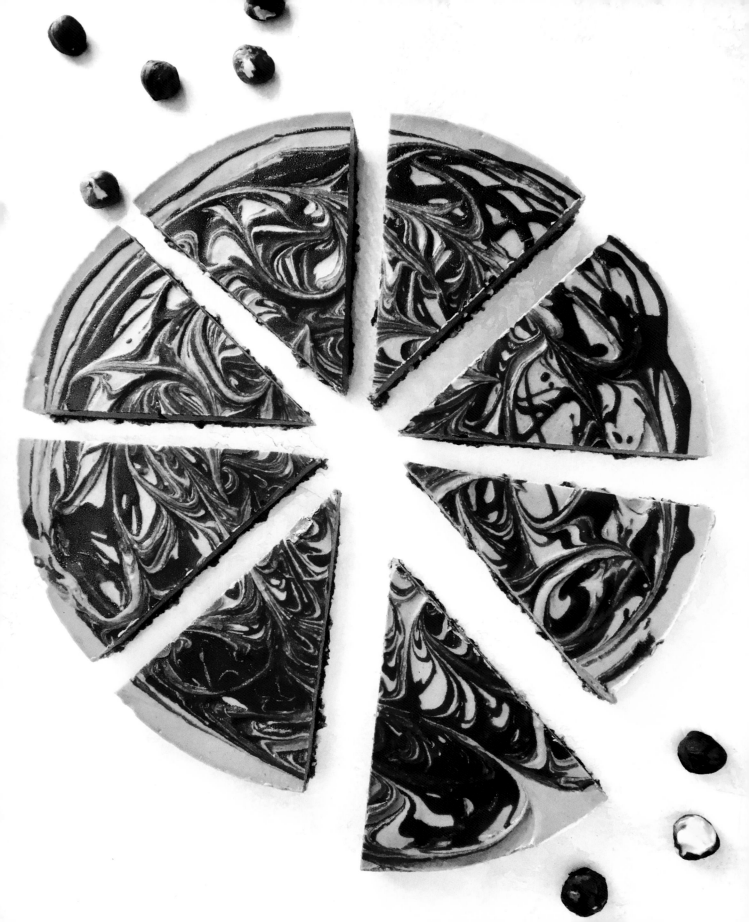

Chocolate Hazelnut Cheesecake

MAKES ONE 9-INCH CHEESECAKE

Our daughter, Savannah, loves healthy food, but before she went completely plant based, her guilty pleasure was Nutella. It is no mystery why this chocolaty, nutty, creamy, sweet, and salty spread is so widely used in Europe and the United States. It is something that can easily convert a nonbeliever into a complete sweet-tooth fanatic. With this recipe, Tamal set out to take that same chocolate and hazelnut goodness and morph it into a cheesecake concept. This dessert is so satisfying and comforting, it'll transport you—by way of taste receptors—to Italy to dance around the Colosseum! In all seriousness, everyone who loves nuts and chocolate will enjoy this decadent treat.

For the oven-roasted hazelnuts

1½ cups raw hazelnuts

1   Preheat the oven to 350 degrees F.

2   Roast the hazelnuts on a dry baking sheet for 10–12 minutes, or until their skin starts to come off, the nuts are cracking, and their color turns a light golden brown.

3   Remove the hazelnuts from the oven, place on a clean, dry towel, and rub them vigorously to get as much skin off as you can.

4   Divide the hazelnuts in half, reserving ¾ cup for the crust and ¾ cup for the filling.

To make an optional chocolate garnish, melt 1 Tbsp. coconut oil and 3 Tbsp. vegan chocolate chips in a small pan over low heat. Drizzle the chocolate over the cheesecake before freezing.

▶

Chocolate Hazelnut Cheesecake (*cont.*)

For the crust

1 cup salted macadamia nuts

¾ cup oven-roasted hazelnuts

1 Tbsp. cocoa powder

¾ cup pitted dates
(preferably Medjool)

½ tsp. vanilla extract

1 tsp. extra-virgin coconut oil

1. In a food processor, blitz the salted macadamia nuts, roasted hazelnuts, and cocoa powder until fine granules form.

2. Add the dates, vanilla extract, and extra-virgin coconut oil. Blend until the mixture forms a grainy dough.

3. Press the crust mixture into a 9-inch cheesecake pan with your fingers. Let it set in the freezer while you make the filling.

For the filling

¾ cup oven-roasted hazelnuts

¾ cup water

1 cup soaked cashews

½ cup coconut cream

½ cup coconut oil

½ cup pitted dates
(preferably Medjool)

3 Tbsp. cocoa powder

2 Tbsp. maple syrup

½ tsp. vanilla extract

⅛ tsp. Himalayan pink salt

1 tsp. sunflower lecithin

1. Place the roasted hazelnuts in a high-powered blender with ¾ cup water and blitz for 45 seconds.

2. Pour the mixture into a cheesecloth set over a bowl. Squeeze as much milk out as possible with your hands. You should get at least ½ cup hazelnut milk through this process. Discard the pulp.

3. Place the hazelnut milk and the rest of the filling ingredients into a high-powered blender. Blitz twice for 45 seconds each time, or until creamy smooth.

4. Pour the filling into the cheesecake pan. Let set in the freezer for 1 hour.

Going Bananas Cream Pie

There are some classic desserts that can't be left behind, so we have to create a healthy, scrumptious spin on them. That way, we get all of the delicious flavor without the negative side effects from poor ingredients. This Going Bananas Cream Pie won't sit for long—it's irresistible. We might say you'll go bananas for it!

For the crust

1 cup pecans

1 cup macadamia nuts

⅓ cup chopped pitted dates (preferably Medjool)

Pinch of Himalayan pink salt

1   Place pecans and macadamia nuts in a food processor and blitz until the pieces are the size of quinoa gains or short-grain brown rice.

2   Add in the chopped dates and salt. Blitz until mixed well.

3   Pour the crust mixture into a 9-inch pie pan and press down evenly with your fingers until you have covered the bottom. Place in the freezer to chill while you work on the filling.

For the filling

1 cup raw cashews, soaked for at least 2 hours

1 13.5-oz. can coconut cream, chilled overnight or for at least 2 hours

2 bananas

¼ cup coconut oil

2 Tbsp. lemon juice

¼ cup maple syrup

½ tsp. vanilla extract

Pinch of Himalayan pink salt

Juice from 1 lime

1   Place the cashews into a high-powered blender or food processor.

2   Without shaking it, open the can of coconut cream. Drain out the water and use *only* the cream. Add the coconut cream to the blender or food processor with 1 banana, coconut oil, lemon juice, maple syrup, vanilla extract, and salt. Blitz twice for 45 seconds each time, or until smooth.

3   Pour the filling into the crust. Cover with plastic wrap and place in the freezer for at least 2 hours to set.

4   While the pie sets, slice the second banana into a bowl and cover the pieces in the lime juice. Use the banana slices to garnish the top of your pie before serving.

Salty Chocolate Peanut Butter Bars

MAKES ONE 9x5 LOAF PAN

Candy tastes delicious. That is why millions of people eat it every day. When it comes to feeding our children sweets, though, we educate them about why sugar, dyes, and preservatives are bad for your body. We let our kids know that candy isn't a good choice. On the flip side, we don't want our children to feel left out, and we want them to enjoy delicious desserts. So we make healthy alternatives to store-bought junk food. These Salty Chocolate Peanut Butter Bars are so nutritious that even adults won't hesitate to indulge. They'll cure anyone's sweet-tooth craving.

½ cup salted peanuts

½ cup salted macadamia nuts

½ cup pitted dates (preferably Medjool)

½ tsp. vanilla extract

1 cup salted peanut butter

½ cup coconut sugar

4 Tbsp. coconut oil

⅛ tsp. Himalayan pink salt

2 Tbsp. coconut flour

½ tsp. vanilla extract

¼ cup brown rice cereal, such as One Degree

¼ cup vegan chocolate chips

1 Line the bottom and sides of a 9x5 loaf pan with parchment paper.

2 Place the salted peanuts and macadamia nuts in a food processor and blitz until the nuts reach a crumb consistency.

3 Add the dates and vanilla extract and blitz again until a dough-like consistency is formed. Press this mixture with your hands into the parchment paper-lined pan. It should be about ½ inch thick and evenly spread. Let set in the freezer while you make the filling.

4 In a medium-size bowl, combine the peanut butter, coconut sugar, 3 Tbsp. coconut oil, salt, coconut flour, and vanilla extract and mix well. Add in the brown rice cereal and mix until combined.

5 Remove the crust from the freezer and spoon in the filling, spreading it evenly over the crust. Return the pan to the freezer.

6 In a small pan over low heat, melt together the chocolate chips and remaining 1 Tbsp. coconut oil.

7 Remove the pan from the freezer again and drizzle the chocolate over the bars in a pattern or pour the chocolate on and spread evenly over the top, depending on the look you are going for. Return the bars to the freezer for at least 2 hours before serving.

8 When you are ready to serve, pull out the parchment paper, and the whole block of bars should come out easily. To cut into squares smoothly, use a large knife that has been warmed under hot water and dried.

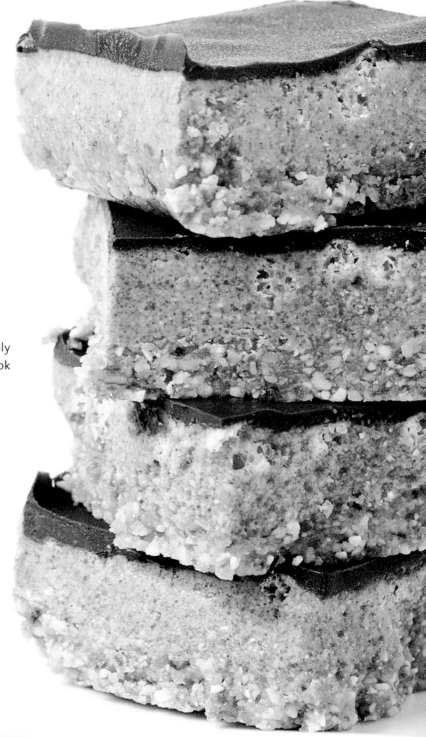

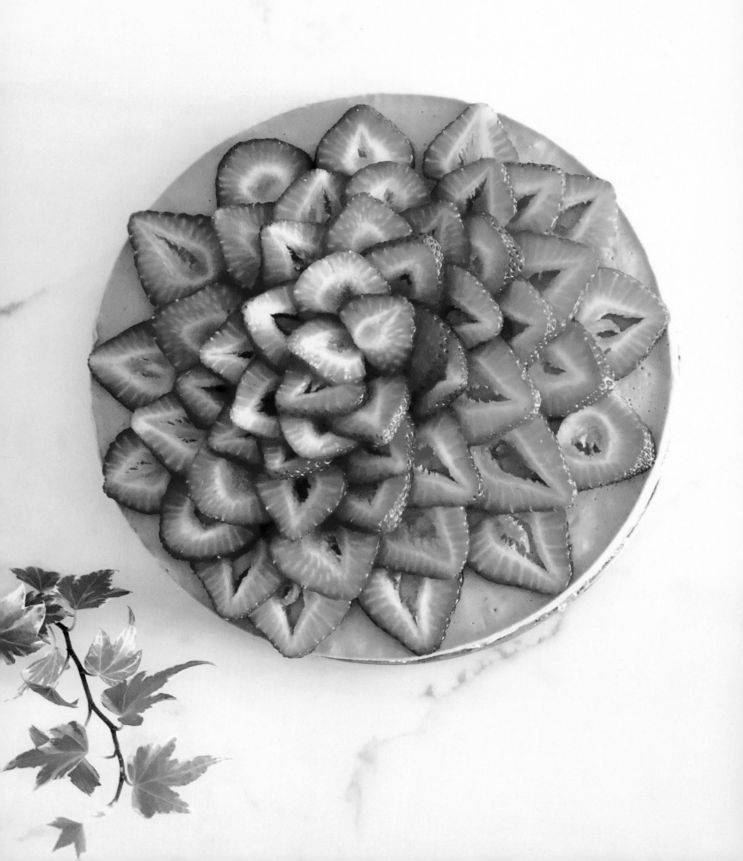

Strawberry Cheesecake with Macadamia Nut Crust

Cheesecake is special to Tamal. His mother was a master of desserts and plant-based cuisine. He remembers his mother showing him how to design each cheesecake, including all sorts of tricks to make them taste and look appealing. Tamal has spent countless hours crafting different cheesecake staples to please even the toughest critic of plant-based versions of dairy sweets. This Strawberry Cheesecake has been requested countless times for family gatherings, parties, and birthdays! We have yet to find someone who doesn't want to eat the whole thing.

For the crust

½ cup walnuts

½ cup salted macadamia nuts

½ cup dates (preferably Medjool)

1 tsp. lemon zest

1 Place the nuts in a food processor and blitz till they reach a crumb-like texture, around 10–15 seconds.

2 Add dates and lemon zest into the nut mixture in the food processor and blend until the dates and nuts are like small crumbs.

3 Spoon the crust mixture into an 8-inch cheesecake pan. Pat the crust down with your fingers so that it covers the bottom of the pan. It's fine if it looks a bit messy, as the filling will cover it up. Let it set in the freezer while you work on the filling.

▶

Strawberry Cheesecake with Macadamia Nut Crust *(cont.)*

For the filling

1½ cups raw cashews, soaked

½ cup coconut cream, chilled overnight or for at least for 2 hours

2 Tbsp. lemon juice

¼ cup melted coconut oil

¼ cup maple syrup

⅛ tsp. Himalayan pink salt

½ tsp. lemon zest

½ cup fresh or frozen and thawed strawberries

¼ tsp. vanilla extract

1 Place all the filling ingredients in a high-powered blender or food processor and blitz twice for 45 seconds each time, or until creamy smooth, like a cheesecake filling.

2 Remove the crust from the freezer. Pour the filling mixture into the crust. Smooth it out with a spoon or spatula.

3 Place strawberries as garnish on top or press them into the cheesecake filling.

4 Freeze the cheesecake for at least 1–2 hours to set. Store in the refrigerator.

Country-Style Strawberry Rhubarb Crumble

MAKES ONE 9x9-INCH PAN

It isn't easy to strike the right balance of sweetness and tartness with a rhubarb crumble. We worked hard, trying a variety of approaches, before we got it just right. This recipe will please rhubarb novices and crumble connoisseurs alike! Country-Style Strawberry Rhubarb Crumble pairs deliciously with coconut whipped cream or vegan ice cream.

For the topping

¾ cup white whole-wheat pastry flour

¾ cup rolled oats

¼ tsp. Himalayan pink salt

¼ cup coconut sugar

½ tsp. cinnamon

¼ tsp. baking powder

¼ cup plus 1 Tbsp. melted coconut oil

1. Preheat the oven to 375 degrees F.

2. Mix all the dry topping ingredients together until well combined.

3. Add in the coconut oil and mix to form a slightly moist crumble. Set aside while you prepare the filling.

For the filling

3 cups rhubarb (sliced into ¼-inch pieces)

3 cups strawberries (sliced into ¼-inch pieces)

¾ cup coconut sugar

2 Tbsp. white whole-wheat pastry flour

3 Tbsp. arrowroot powder

½ tsp. cinnamon

¼ tsp. Himalayan pink salt

2 tsp. lemon juice

1. In a large bowl, stir together the chopped rhubarb, strawberries, coconut sugar, flour, arrowroot powder, cinnamon, salt, and lemon juice until well combined.

2. Pour the filling mixture into a 9x9-inch pan and cover with the topping.

3. Bake the crumble in the oven for 35 minutes, or until the top is golden brown and the filling is bubbly.

The Peanut Butter Cup

MAKES ABOUT 1 DOZEN 2-INCH CUPS

Many of us remember eating Reese's peanut butter cups when we were children. That combination of sweet, salty, creamy, and nutty is pure perfection! This recipe was inspired by Tamal's love of peanut butter and chocolate. He wanted to make something that tastes like a favorite childhood candy but also embodies an adult's wisdom about health and wellness. We like to use grain- or stevia-sweetened vegan chocolate chips. This mouthwatering peanut butter cup is satisfying and nourishing.

½ cup salted creamy peanut butter

4 Tbsp. coconut sugar

1 tsp. coconut flour

⅛ tsp. Himalayan pink salt

1½ Tbsp. extra-virgin coconut oil

1½ cups vegan chocolate chips

1 In a large bowl, mix together the peanut butter, coconut sugar, coconut flour, and salt until well combined.

2 In a small pot over low heat, melt together the coconut oil and chocolate chips, stirring continuously so the mixture doesn't burn. It should take 2–3 minutes and result in a smooth mixture, like a chocolate sauce.

3 Using a 2-inch nonstick silicone chocolate mold, fill it one-third of the way with the chocolate mixture, another third of the way with the peanut butter mixture, and the last third with more chocolate. Repeat this process until you have filled your dozen molds and used up all the chocolate and peanut butter mixtures.

4 Let the peanut butter cups set in the freezer for 2 hours before serving.

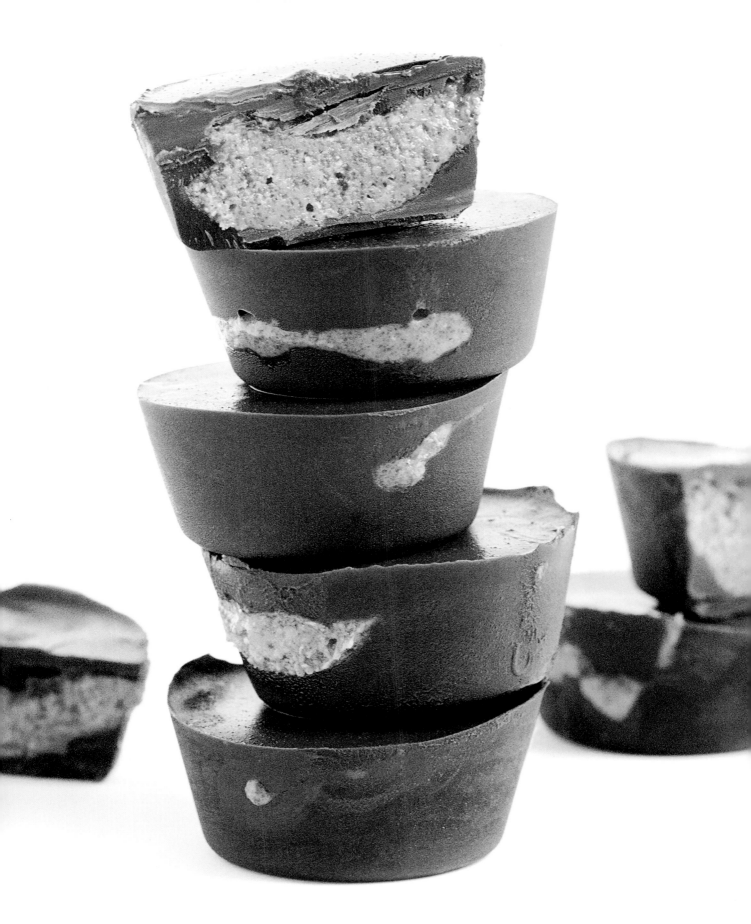

Key Lime Cheesecake

MAKES ONE 9-INCH PIE

Key lime pie is one of the most popular dishes in America. It is sweet, tart, and rich. That flavor combination translates perfectly to cheesecakes. We have created a Key Lime Cheesecake that is so decadent and fulfilling, it'll win over any pie or cheesecake lover in a heartbeat. Plus it is packed with superfoods and other healthy ingredients. The avocado is the star in this recipe. It gives the cheesecake a beautiful green color and adds a creaminess that is amazing in flavor and depth. This delicious dessert will satisfy your body as well as your sweet tooth.

For the crust

1 cup pecans

1 cup walnuts

1 tsp. coconut oil

½ cup pitted dates
(preferably Medjool)

⅛ tsp. Himalayan pink salt

½ tsp. vanilla extract

1 Place the pecans and walnuts in a food processor and blend until the nut pieces are small and granular, about the size of rice grains.

2 Add the coconut oil, dates, salt, and vanilla extract to the food processor. Blitz until the mixture forms a crust-like consistency.

3 Spoon the crust into a 9-inch cheesecake pan. Press the mixture into the base of the pan evenly with your fingers. Set the pan in the freezer while you work on the filling.

For best results, chill a can of coconut milk overnight in the refrigerator to use in this recipe.

For the filling

1 cup raw cashews, soaked
for at least 2 hours

½ cup chilled coconut milk

½ cup coconut oil

½ cup maple syrup

¼ cup fresh-squeezed lime juice

½ tsp. vanilla extract

½ cup avocado chunks

Pinch of Himalayan pink salt

1 Place all the of the ingredients except the avocado into a high-powered blender and blitz on high for 45 seconds, or until creamy and smooth.

2 Separate ¼ cup of the filling mixture and set aside. Add the avocado chunks to the rest of the mixture in the blender and blitz again for 45 seconds, or until creamy and smooth.

3 Pour the avocado mixture into the cheesecake pan and spread evenly. Tap the pan lightly on a cutting board to get out any air bubbles.

4 Drizzle the reserved ¼ cup white mixture all over the top of the green cheesecake, as if you are trying to draw lines with it. With a toothpick tip, carefully swirl the lines to create the classic cheesecake look.

5 Place in the freezer for at least 2 hours to set. About 15 minutes before serving, remove from the freezer. To get perfectly clean slices, run your knife under hot water before cutting each piece.

6 Store in an airtight container in the refrigerator for up to 1 week or in the freezer for about 3 weeks.

Metric Conversions

BY VOLUME

Imperial	Metric
½ teaspoon	2.5 milliliters
1 teaspoon	5 milliliters
1 tablespoon	15 milliliters
¼ cup	60 milliliters
⅓ cup	80 milliliters
½ cup	120 milliliters
⅔ cup	160 milliliters
¾ cup	180 milliliters
1 cup	240 milliliters

BY WEIGHT

Imperial	Metric
1 ounce	28 grams
¼ pound	113 grams
½ pound	227 grams
¾ pound	340 grams
1 pound	454 grams

BY LENGTH

Imperial	Metric
1 inch	2.5 centimeters
6 inches	15 centimeters
12 inches	30 centimeters

OVEN TEMPERATURES

Fahrenheit	Celsius
300 degrees F	150 degrees C
325 degrees F	165 degrees C
350 degrees F	180 degrees C
375 degrees F	190 degrees C
400 degrees F	200 degrees C
425 degrees F	220 degrees C
450 degrees F	230 degrees C
475 degrees F	245 degrees C

acknowledgments

It takes a lot of hands on deck to create something meaningful and worthwhile. This book wouldn't exist without the generosity and help of the many people who stepped in to make it happen. First, we want to thank our dear friend and mentor Kathy Hoshijo: without your continual guidance and leadership, we wouldn't be here. To our friends and family who spent countless hours being force-fed good and bad recipes during our testing phase: because of your resilience and love, we now have a book filled with 108 delicious recipes. This project would never have happened without Liz Arch, our colleague, friend, and a beautiful soul. Your belief in our idea and your generosity have made this concept into a reality. To our incredible agent, Coleen O'Shea: your insight, dedication, and professionalism are nothing short of inspiring. To our publishers at Sounds True: you guys rock, and your vision for this book goes far beyond our wildest expectations. We are honored to be working with you. To our children, Savannah and Kanai, and anyone we may have missed, we thank you from the bottom of our hearts!

index

about the authors

TAMAL DODGE was born and raised in his family's yoga ashram in Hawaii and has been teaching and practicing yoga since childhood. Tamal is the founder of Yoga Salt, one of the most popular yoga centers in Los Angeles, and has been featured in *TIME* magazine, *Los Angeles Times*, *New York Times*, *Chicago Tribune*, Reuters, MSNBC, *Self* magazine, *Yogi Times*, *Better Homes and Gardens*, Martha Stewart Living Radio, FitTV, and numerous other national and international media.

Tamal has several best-selling yoga DVDs, including *Hatha and Flow Yoga for Beginners*, *Yoga for Energy and Relaxation*, and *Intro to Yoga*, all of which are currently sold worldwide. Tamal also tours the country teaching workshops, seminars, conferences, and yoga teacher trainings to the masses. Tamal's goal is to help people be "in the world but not of the world," to become truly peaceful and happy, and to make yoga a lifestyle. For more, please visit yogasalt.com.

VICTORIA DODGE is a professional photographer who has worked with Lululemon, *Forbes* magazine, Oscar-winning director James Cameron, and athlete and wellness advocate Rich Roll. As a cooking expert, she has taught the likes of *This Is Us* star Sterling K. Brown and supermodel Lindsey Wixon. Additionally, Victoria is the founder of *The Yoga Plate* blog, which has featured interviews with such best-selling authors as Mimi Kirk, John Robbins, and Seane Corn. Find more of her work at theyogaplate.com.

about sounds true

Sounds True is a multimedia publisher whose mission is to inspire and support personal transformation and spiritual awakening. Founded in 1985 and located in Boulder, Colorado, we work with many of the leading spiritual teachers, thinkers, healers, and visionary artists of our time. We strive with every title to preserve the essential "living wisdom" of the author or artist. It is our goal to create products that not only provide information to a reader or listener, but that also embody the quality of a wisdom transmission.

For those seeking genuine transformation, Sounds True is your trusted partner. At SoundsTrue.com you will find a wealth of free resources to support your journey, including exclusive weekly audio interviews, free downloads, interactive learning tools, and other special savings on all our titles.

To learn more, please visit SoundsTrue.com/freegifts or call us toll-free at 800.333.9185.

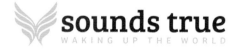